Niblet and The Great Additive Caper

Marshall Carder

ISBN: 0615745946
ISBN-13: 978-0615745947

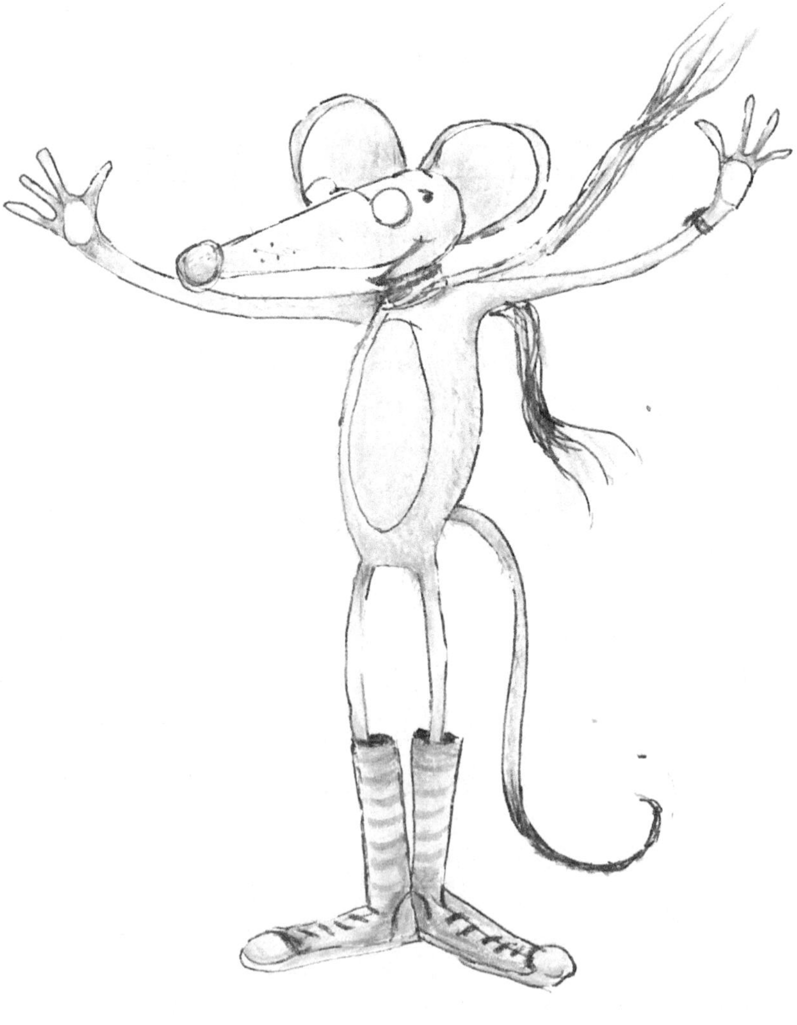

DEDICATION

This book is the culmination of thirty years in the food industry and fourteen years of parenthood. It is the conversation about food I believe every parent should have with their children, and themselves. While I am not a scientist, I have spent my life working in the food industry, cooking every day and trying to maintain good health in this crazy world that is food today. I read voraciously and feel the need to share what I have learned.

I dedicate this book to my wife and my children, who are my inspiration, along with my family and friends, too many to name. To know me is to know my passion for food, family, friends, music and most of all, great conversation.

This is one I share with you.

Cover Art By Pat Carder-Senecal – Interior Picture of Niblet by Lee Lorgus

CONTENTS

	Acknowledgments	i
1	The Book	1
2	Niblet	3
3	Wesa	9
4	The Mystery	13
5	The Escape	23
6	Mission To The Pantry	32
7	Identifying the Worst Ingredients	50
8	Breaking Down the Label	79
9	Shouting From the Hills	106
10	Times Have Changed	125

SPECIAL DE-CODER PAGE AT VERY END

ACKNOWLEDGMENTS

Special thanks go to my Mother, Father and daughter Giuliana who helped me articulate this book, and to Ana and Olivia who believed in my vision. Thanks also to Ellen Burke and Amy Carey for the invaluable editing assistance.

1 THE BOOK

Perhaps the word "nutcase" might be a little strong, but Professor B's colleagues had changed the way they spoke about him ever since that old crazy mouse incident all those years back. He took it all in stride and never let his confidence or conviction waver, but life at the University just wasn't the same since then. He had gone out and worked in industrial science and made his mark, but now back on Campus all anyone remembered was the mouse. And, yet, "That mouse had changed the world after all," he reflected, so it figured that everyone would still be talking about it. Professor B knew deep down that it was worth every bit of trouble that it had caused him, and sure enough he would do it again if he had the chance; even if nobody could get past that crazy story.

Giuliana and Olivia, his grandkids, really had experienced quite an adventure when they set out to help their African friend Wesa. He was suffering from poor health and malaise just a few months after coming to live in the United States. Nobody would have predicted just how this story unfolded. "Good thing the kids got it down on paper," he said aloud to himself.

He chuckled as he opened the book Wesa had just finished writing about the whole fiasco. The girls had helped fill in all the little details. "Well here it is, after all, laid bare for all to see," he thought. He hoped they remembered everything he had told them, but deep down he knew they had. Wesa and Giuliana didn't miss much, that was for sure, and if they did, little ole' Olivia was right there to remind them, over and over and over, with some kind of goofy face on, as was her way. "This is going to be fun," he thought.

Professor B got up from his chair to freshen his cup from the teapot in the corner, the newly printed book stuffed under his arm. Then he walked toward the window and looked out, down towards the community garden below that was teaming with fresh vegetables and herbs. "Things really can change if you stick to your convictions, keep your head up, and never give up the fight," he mumbled aloud. "That garden used to be a perfectly manicured and perfectly useless lawn that nobody was even allowed to walk on. Now it provided fresh produce and brought the neighborhood together to boot. But more, it was a symbol of what can happen when you believe in change…and have the courage to listen to a little mouse," he smiled. He sat down again in his comfy chair next to the window and opened the book to the first page, and with great anticipation, he began to read.

2 NIBLET

Down in the laboratory, just past all those bubbling flasks of who knows what, Professor B had a small office. While not much to look at, and certainly not the envy of his peers, the office afforded Professor B the best view of everything going on in the Lab, and it kept him close to Niblet.

Niblet had seemed like a very special mouse from the very first time Professor B saw him, but he wasn't exactly sure why. After all, he looked identical to all of the other mice. But there was this special way that he looked at Professor B that had saved it in the end. Professor B had taken Niblet from the mouse population destined for the studies and experiments in the lab and had created a nice space for him in the corner of the office, down in the basement. Professor B had grown tired of subjecting the poor little mice to all of the prodding and poking and injecting and measuring and what not. Yeah, he knew much of it was important to the Company; he had just lost his heart for the work. So he had retreated to the old lab in the basement to see if he could just figure out what that little mouse was trying to tell him. And boy would he be surprised.

Professor B began with the usual communication techniques. He introduced symbols, signs, and even words to the mouse. He created a special set of computer programs that would help the mouse learn his letters and sounds. And then, just when he felt that Niblet was starting to get it, his hopes would be dashed by a battery of testing gone bad. But he didn't give up because he just knew that little brain was humming along nicely. Somehow he could tell. You know, the way that you can sometimes read a face from a distance, regardless of the country or language, and know exactly what the person is trying to say? Well Professor B knew that Niblet was going to speak to him one day.. It was just a matter of time.

Every day Professor B came to the office and dreamed up new ways to teach the mouse something. And slowly but surely he felt he was seeing progress. It seemed clear to him that the mouse was beginning to understand, but they still had no reliable or quick way for Niblet to communicate back. Oh, Professor B thought of many things. He even used sensors to try to amplify the mouse vocals only to discover the problems with whole ranges of sounds that the mouse simply couldn't make.

One day, after sending email on his little smart device thingee, Professor B laid it on his desk, and went to check if the new sensors he had ordered were in. He didn't really like to be bothered trudging all of the way upstairs, but the mail department would only deliver them at the end of the day and he wanted to push forward with his latest idea. Niblet was sitting on the desk in front of the computer and seemed entirely absorbed in the new mathematics software that Professor B had just put on, so he left him there on the table.

And that was Niblet's chance! He was going to finally show Professor B what he had learned. He had mustered the courage, he had been thinking. "I shouldn't have done so poorly on those tests," he lamented "It wasn't fair to Professor B." But he was kind of scared to come out and start communicating, and he really didn't have a reliable way to do that yet anyway. He was naturally very shy after all, so he had failed the tests on purpose. But over time, Niblet had grown to love Professor B and now he really wanted to show what he had learned. So as soon as the professor left, Niblet scurried over to the smart phone lying on the desk. The keyboard was still too big for him, but much easier to handle than the laptop. He had to jump around on the huge keyboards and so he typed very slowly and he made mistakes so it really didn't work well at all. He had never gotten his hands on the Professor's smart phone but that little keyboard looked far easier to handle.

He tapped the screen several times, and opened up a new email message, just like he had seen the Professor do so many times from atop his shoulder. Hmm, "Who should I write to?" He thought. "I got it."

There was this other man who was always making fun of Professor B's attempts to educate a mouse. Niblet thought his name was Johnson or something. He began to type, J.O.H.N and the program pulled up a name, Johnson.David@cclp.edu. "That must be it," Niblet thought and selected the name. "Let's start slowly. How about this," he typed "If you can read this message, then you're wrong about mice. Signed, Niblet."

"Ok, now let's see. Where do I? Oh yeah, that's right, SEND!" he remembered, and off the message went. Nobody could have figured exactly how much that email would change Professor B's life, especially not Niblet, but away it went.

Dr. Johnson had felt that it was his obligation to speak out regarding Professor B's obsession with the mouse. The Company had given Professor B the time to "do his own work" when he became disenchanted with the other research, due to all of the great science he had produced in the past. But Dr. Johnson and the others were testing the genetically modified foods and all of the "wonderful" new additives and colors the Company was making and saw no reason why Professor B should not be applying his great mind to the task at hand rather than spending so much Company time and money with that pesky little rodent. The tests were important to the Company bottom line and would help to increase the shelf life and durability of so many of the Company products that Professor B's refusal to conduct further tests incensed Dr. Johnson.

Maybe it was simply jealousy, but in the end Dr. Johnson began one of those whispering campaigns and soon enough the rumors about Professor B that were swirling around were as wild and crazy as they were false. There was nothing that seemed out of the question. Professor B's appearance, his sanity, his past great work which now eluded him were all spoken of, none of which were even close to the truth but went round and round as these things often do. Slowly it began to wear on Professor B and he began to think long and hard about his future in the private sector. But Professor B was a loyal and honorable man. He kept sticking it out because he felt a breakthrough was near with the mouse and that would bring so much good attention and goodwill to the Company that surely those rumors would be dashed once and for all.

Alas, it was exactly Niblet's doing shall we say, that became Professor B's undoing. You see, that email to old Dr. Johnson created an uproar because he steadfastly refused to believe that Niblet had penned it. He initially brought it to Professor B's attention who, obviously, denied authorship. Dr. Johnson then blamed the grandchildren. Certainly "They were the culprits!" he cried. But nope, they were busy at school at the very time the message was sent so it could not be them. Finally, Dr. Johnson brought the matter to the Board, trying to demonstrate that Professor B really was MAD as a hatter after all, and prone to wasting Company time on silly antics like writing emails pretending to be some kind of wonder-mouse.

In the end, all of this became too much for Professor B. Instead of sticking it out and proving all of those naysayers wrong, he chose to rest on his laurels and simply go home. Niblet had become very frightened at the ruckus he had caused, so he never sent another message or made any other indication that he had. Professor B felt there was no use in trying to prove that he was right, because in fact, he was not even sure himself. Instead he went to his office with a small box and packed his personal things.

There wasn't much to take home even though the office was bursting with experimental equipment, measuring devices, projectors, computers and what not. All of this stuff represented his failure with the mouse and he decided it was best to leave it behind. "I'll just go home, give the mouse to the grandchildren and pretend that this last little time I have spent at the Company never actually happened." Professor B was ready to retire from corporate work anyway and there was so much he wanted to do in his garden.

And that is how Giuliana and Olivia came to befriend Niblet. All of the work Professor B had put in with Niblet would prove invaluable to their lives but at the time nobody even knew it.

3 WESA

Sliding along the branch near the top of the tree, Olivia reached the trunk again and let out a sigh of relief. She loved to push her limits and had gotten way out on a very high branch only to realize the only way back was the way she came. She let out a weird sort of yelp, and skooched ever so carefully back toward the trunk of the tree. "All better now," she thought. Giuliana was sitting several branches down near the bottom of the tree, perched gracefully like one of those large cats asleep on the branch, only she wasn't sleeping. She was reading…about 497 pages in and only halfway finished. If there were two things for certain about these two girls, it was that Olivia loved to push her limits and GiuGiu loved to read. Yes, they also shared a passion for LPS and American Girl Dolls, and of course, the guitar, but if they were doing none of those other things it was for sure they were either pushing the envelope, or reading. That was their way.

This day was special because it was the first time they were to see Wesa in person. They had heard so much about him before he came from Africa and they had been texting and emailing since he got here but things had been so busy that they had not yet met him in person although it had already been several months since his arrival.

Wesa was from a very small village in Angola. As an infant, his parents were lost in a terrible accident. He had been brought to an orphanage where he was cared for by Sister D. One day, this great American family that had been working there for one of the big petroleum companies decided to adopt him. The wife had been helping Sister D with fundraising and office stuff and had fallen in love with Wesa. He was such a smart and energetic boy. He could outrun all of the kids in the school even though many were years older. He loved to study and learn even when it was hard. Yeah, he complained a bit, but then got right back to work. He was everything a parent could want in a child.

Olivia spotted him first. Of course, she was way up in the top of the tree and Giuliana's face was still buried in her book anyway, so it really was no contest. Olivia knew he would be happy to see them and she began to quack like a duck using her hands to make the bird call, "Quaaak, Quaack," she squawked .

Wesa heard the noise and looked up toward the tree. "Sounds like a pretty funny bird," he thought. "Quaak Quaak, Wesa," Olivia said again. He looked back toward the tree and now he could make something out. It was Giuliana leaning back on the branch, finally looking up from her book. "Giuliana," Wesa cried aloud. "Wesa," both of the girls said together. "Jinx, Jinx, double jinx" they went on. "…stop it!" Olivia demanded. "Let's get down from this…" and without even finishing her sentence she swung down from the tree and landed in front of, almost on top of actually,

Wesa. Giuliana gracefully slid from the tree with one hand while the other secured the book, certain to hold her page with one finger. They smiled. They beamed. They were so happy to see Wesa, but he seemed a bit off to them. Yeah, he smiled and hugged them but something was amiss. In fact, Wesa didn't look exactly the same as the pictures they had exchanged with him, and he didn't even climb the tree and he was known for that.

"I heard you were the fastest kid in the orphanage," Giuliana began.

"Uh, yeah I guess I was." said Wesa.

"Well I'm not so slow myself. I'll race you to the end of the park and back," said Giuliana. "I'm in too." said Olivia and she dashed off toward the turnaround point by the water fountain. Giuliana was not going to let her get too far ahead so she looked at Wesa and shouted, "Come on, last one is a rotten egg." Wesa turned and ran but Giuliana was out in front of him and he simply couldn't close the gap. He did manage to catch up with Olivia, but she was much younger. He felt sort of sad and defeated but just near the finish line Giuliana slowed way down and said, "Come on Wesa! Come on Olivia! We can finish together and nobody will be a rotten egg."

Wesa was relieved that he had saved face a bit, but he felt he needed to tell the girls what was happening to him. Ever since he had moved in with the new family his body and his mind had begun to change. And unfortunately it was not for the better. "Look Giuliana, I know you are fast but I can barely keep up with Olivia. I just don't feel right, I don't have the right energy, and worse, I am having a hard time concentrating and keeping up with my studies."

The girls were very sad to hear this and asked Wesa if he had told his parents about what was going on, and of course he had. His parents were very loving and caring and had brought Wesa to the best doctors.

They had told him he needed more exercise and had recommended some pills that his parents could give him to help him concentrate. It was OK to take these pills the Doctor had told him, because it was very common these days. But Wesa did not like pills at all, and he did not feel like exercising, he just felt like sitting on the couch and eating because he needed the calories for energy. This was not what the girls wanted to hear at all.

"Well this is very interesting," said Olivia.

"Yes, in fact it is very mysterious. How could a perfectly healthy, happy and smart young man fall into such a state in such a short period of time," said Giuliana. "You have only been here for six months, right Wesa?"

"Dahn, dahn, daahn…" said Olivia, trying to create a soundtrack for Giuliana's mystery.

"Well I say we go speak with my Dad and get a couple of clues that we might go on to solve this mystery. Are you in Wesa?"

"Uh, yeah sure. I just have to call my parents and let them know where I am going. I am sure they won't mind." said Wesa.

So Wesa called his parents, and off the three of them went, through the narrow path beside the brook and straight up the hill. They were going to solve this mystery, they were certain. They just were not sure how. Little did they know that Niblet, their yet to be famous Wonder Mouse would provide just the help they needed.

4 THE MYSTERY

Giuliana went straight to the backyard to speak with her father. Although she knew that he was not a doctor and may not have the answer to Wesa's problem, he did always give her something to think about and explore and he always suggested different books for further research.

Dad was busy working on the yard, getting ready for Professor B's retirement party when the three kids came upon him in a rush, the dog never far behind.

"Dad, dad, we need to speak with you," Olivia huffed loudly as she tried to catch her breath.

"Just let me explain," Giuliana implored.

"Hold on, slow down," said Dad calmly, "There will be time for everyone to tell the story, but first, this must be Wesa. Hello Wesa, welcome. How are you?" he continued. Dad set down the hedge cutters, wiped his brow and sat down on the stairs to listen.

"Well, actually, that is what we were coming to speak with you about." said Wesa. "I have not been feeling like myself for some time now and have already gone to the Doctor for examinations. The Doc said I was ok but suggested more exercise and also offered me a pill to help me concentrate. But I never needed these things back in Africa. I ran all of the time just because it was fun, and now I just don't feel like it. I never had problems concentrating either, but now I am ready to take the medicine just to help my studies."

"Wow," Dad exclaimed, "that is quite a story, and not a very happy one I am afraid."

"Yeah it is! And Wesa even lost to Giuliana in a foot race down at the park. From what I heard, I didn't think anyone could beat Wesa." Olivia piped in ecstatically.

"Well," Dad began slowly. "Let's get down to the basics. If you are not feeling well and you don't have a specific disease or sickness it could have to do with what you are putting in your body. You know, the food that you eat can make you sick just as surely as it can make you well. As Hippocrates counseled more than 2,500 years ago, 'Let food be thy medicine and let medicine be thy food. ' All other things being equal and given that your doctor has not found any other causes, we should certainly look first at what you are eating, because the solution to your problem might be that simple. What would happen to your father's fine automobile if he put the wrong fuel in the tank?" Dad spoke rhetorically.

"Hey, before we go any further, let's go inside and get out of the hot sun. Wouldn't you guys like some nice cold lemonade?"

Dad asked. "Why don't you come inside and we'll talk further over a frosty beverage. I definitely like a good mystery, especially when it involves food. I have a good feeling that we can solve it for you Wesa." Dad added.

Dad got up and grabbed his shirt, putting it on as he walked toward the house. Upstairs in the kitchen the air was a bit cooler and there was a great big jar of fresh lemonade in the fridge. The lemon tree had really boomed this year and they were Meyer Lemons, a very sweet variety that produced excellent lemonade. The kids followed Dad up the stairs and sat down in the dining room. He grabbed several glasses and Olivia quickly ran to the fridge to grab the jar of lemonade. She brought the jar to the table and only lost a few drops along the way. She carefully poured four glasses and then sat back and enjoyed the refreshing drink.

"This is the life," she quipped.

"Funny, Olivia." Giuliana scoffed.

"Wesa, I think we need to have a conversation about food." said Dad in a more somber tone.

"Will that really help?" asked Wesa sheepishly.

"You know it will Wesa!" Olivia shouted.

"Giuliana, can you tell Wesa what the rules are for eating in this house?" asked Dad.

"Sure. First I guess we have to start with the fact that most wholesome and healthy food is very easy to recognize. That is, unless it comes in a package or box." said Giuliana. "The closer our foods are to the way they came from the garden or the field, the more certain we can be that we are eating real food and not other things that purport to be food, you know, like all of those crazy snacks your parents put in your lunch. They may have started out as staple crops but they are a long way from that now."

"And, you are saying that we should always try to eat food if we can, I guess?" Wesa asked sheepishly.

"Of course we should be eating food, what else would we eat, snails?" said Olivia.

"Olivia, firstly, technically speaking snails are food, at least in France; however what I am saying is many things that are presented as food and that are in food actually are not food at all," responded Giuliana curtly.

"That is gross, but do tell!" Olivia chirped.

"Yes," said Dad, "These non-foods are what Michael Pollan calls, "Food-Like Substances". These processed foods can look and taste amazing but they are mostly stripped of the fiber, minerals, vitamins and other nutrients that nature originally provided."

"Do you mean they are putting things that are not food in my food? Such as bugs and stuff?" gasped Olivia.

"It's true actually, but insects would be the least of your worries. The real problems lie with the plethora of chemical and artificial additives that are being used," cautioned Giuliana. "Many of the ingredients used in processed foods today are not added for your health or any other actual consumer benefit. In fact, the artificial ingredients are used to make the food looks pretty, smell good and last a million years on the Big Box shelf without degrading in any way. Cool huh? Crazy as it may sound Wesa, many additives are very toxic if you eat too much of them."

"What's more, even when you choose the most basic foods, such as simple fruits or vegetables, there can be residues of synthetic petroleum pesticides and herbicides. Wax, dyes and other chemicals are also added to create better appearance on the shelves. Since many Americans make their food choices with their eyes instead of their brains, industry gives them things that look picture perfect, regardless of the content," said Dad.

"Wait, wait, so let me ask you a question. How do I know that the foods that I choose do not contain these synthetic and harmful chemicals and additives?" asked Wesa.

"Well, with vegetables and fruits, we buy things that are certified organic. This means that the crops have been grown without synthetic chemical pesticides and herbicides. They have also been proven to contain more nutrients. Studies at both UC Davis and Rutgers University have shown this to be true. BUT, we can't rely just on the "organic" label to make our choices, because you can make junk food with organic ingredients. So if we are buying "unprocessed" foods like apples and bananas, the "organic" distinction is what we rely on, but if the food has been processed and packaged what do we have to do?" Dad asked the girls.

"Gotta read the ingreeeeeeeedients." Olivia sang loudly. "If you can't read it or pronounce it, it probably isn't food."

Giuliana jumped in, "If the ingredients sound like a science project then it probably is. Grandma didn't need any of those fancy-shmancy, new-fangled ingredients and she was the best cook around."

"Does all of this make sense to you Wesa?" Dad queried softly.

"I think so. What you are saying is that the mystery of my poor health could be answered when we find out what I am eating?" Wesa asked. "I mean, maybe all of those bright boxes in my pantry are not actually foods at all and I must read the ingredients in order to really know what I am eating? Is that what you are saying?"

"That about sums it up Wesa. Sooooooooo… the question now begs to be asked. What are you eating?" said Giuliana.

"Just normal stuff that people eat here I guess. I don't really know for sure. But it's really good. It certainly is not the same as I used to eat in the village. It's much easier. Everything comes in bright boxes and cooks very fast. Back in Africa we didn't really have anything that came from packages, we just made everything fresh daily which took time. Our diet back home was very simple and did not taste as amazing as the things my parents cook up in that microwave thing. I don't think I could go back to that Village stuff ever." said Wesa.

"From what I am hearing, it sounds like you're eating a lot of processed foods. Is that right Wesa?" asked Dad.

"I guess so. I just eat what my parents and my friends eat. And these foods taste great. How could there be anything wrong with them? My parents wouldn't buy these things if they weren't healthy, would they?" Wesa whimpered.

"Actually, it is likely that your parents have no idea which ingredients might be harmful. Sadly, they probably don't even read the ingredients at all and simply look at the Nutrient Panel. Today, many foods that used to be made the "old-fashioned way" are now full of chemical additives and preservatives. And further, the food industry has been spending big money to deliberately confuse the unwary like your parents. For instance, a recent industry-sponsored media frenzy was created to convince people that a widely used and oft-vilified sweetener is, in fact, just as good as the old fashioned one. Except that it is not. This was carried out by the makers of this insidious additive despite countless independent studies that have found serious health risks associated with its consumption." said Niblet

"Whoa, whoa, wait…Come on, my parents know what they are eating. What you are saying just can't be true," cried. Wesa.

"Oh, yes it can," said Olivia, "My dad has been studying and observing this like, forever. You know even before I was born. Tell him about the food police in Washington."

"Ok, Olivia. You see Wesa, many people imagine an all-knowing agency in Washington with teams of scientists lined up to test all of the ingredients that are entering the food chain, but in fact that is not correct at all. The truth is that we actually know very little about most of the additives that are entering the food supply each year. The Government agencies routinely rely on testing done by manufacturers, who will always present studies prepared by their own scientists in protection of their profits. The horrifying result is that of the more than 80,000 chemicals in use today, only 200 have been adequately tested for safety when consumed. The manufacturers will tell you it is your "personal responsibility" to eat the right things, at the very same time that they are spending huge sums to confuse you," lamented Dad. "These days, the very agencies tasked with monitoring industry and protecting the consumer are staffed by heads of the very industries that they are supposed to be regulating."

"Sounds like the proverbial fox guarding the hen house, and we know how that went." Giuliana exclaimed.

"What we have right now is equivalent to the wild, wild west in to the food industry. Thousands of chemicals and additives are being added each year with very little oversight and independent safety research. Claims of nutrition and benefits are misleading and confusing and can make it very difficult to know what you are really eating. So in our family we follow some simple rules." Dad continued. "What are they Olivia?"

"Eat foods with as few ingredients as possible." said Olivia

"In other words, you must read the ingredients on everything you eat to know what it is made from. If you can't recognize or understand an ingredient, it has probably been added for some reason other than your better health. Is the ingredient there to preserve, to color, or to moisten? Who cares, because you don't need it and humankind did fine without it for millennia."

"Let me clarify something Wesa. Many people only read the Nutritional Panel, and not the ingredient declaration. However, the nutrient panel will not actually tell you what is in the package. Since not all fats are the same, and not all carbohydrates are the same, and not all proteins are the same and not all sugars are the same, you must always read the ingredients to know for sure what you are eating," Dad continued.

"Wait, wait," Wesa cried. "This is too much for me to believe. Do I really have to know all of this in order get healthy again? Isn't there somebody making sure there aren't bad things in the food. This cannot be true."

"Well Wesa, it is complicated. Unfortunately, the packages are full of promises but you just can't believe them all. You have to read and educate yourself on the basics. But don't worry, you will learn and we will help you. You have no chance of getting good grades or being an athlete unless you fuel yourself properly, which means eating whole foods as much as possible and staying away from artificial and synthetic ingredients. And rest assured Wesa, we're going to make sure that you do." Dad said.

"First we must start with a reading list," and Dad began to list some authors, "Colin Campbell, Dean Ornish, Michael Pollan, Eric Schossler, Marian Nestle. These should help get you started. They will give you an idea just how far from the farm and field we have actually come so that you can begin to restore your health by improving your diet."

In the corner, all the while, quietly sitting in his cage, Niblet was listening to everything that was being discussed. "This is just what I have been waiting for," he thought. Wesa and the girls need to learn about all of these ingredients and I am going to help them. Every one of my relatives were involved in additive testing, and Professor B taught me exactly what happened. But first, I need to read the books that Dad recommended because Professor B never gave me those."

5 THE ESCAPE

So, it came to be that Giuliana and Olivia had gotten the mouse they had always wanted, and Professor B got more time to work in his garden. The girls played and laughed with Niblet, and made him houses and fairy gardens and fed him only organic vegetables and grains. Niblet grew very fond of the two girls as well. At first he had thought they were a little crazy, especially Olivia, but now he understood them much better. The girls had a spirit that you just could not extinguish. Even though their games sometimes got a little out of hand bringing down the "No rough-housing you monkeys!" from the kitchen, they always listened and were mostly well behaved in the end. Niblet dearly wanted to show the kids his special skills, but he was still afraid from all of the commotion he had already caused with Dr. Johnson, so he was very cautious. But, he was getting ready for the day that he would show the world his talent. Then Professor B would be known for his groundbreaking scientific work not just for the fantastic lettuce and cucumbers he grew.

The girls could not be happier with Niblet. Every day after school they would rush home to invent games to play with him. They set up mazes and little play areas, and they carried him around everywhere, often surprising their mother by dropping him on her shoulder when she wasn't looking. This always caused her to shriek loudly when they informed her. Since the kids couldn't understand how anybody could be afraid of Niblet, they just laughed when their mom freaked out. Even the dog, MooMoo loved Niblet. She would sit next to the cage and watch Niblet run on his wheel and climb around. Any chance she got, she would give him a big fat wet loving lick from his head right down to his back. Mom was sure that the dog wanted to eat Niblet, but the kids knew much better. Niblet was family.

"Don't worry mom, MooMoo just loves Niblet. He is one of us now, and MooMoo knows it," Olivia beamed proudly.

Despite all of the reassurances, Mom wasn't entirely convinced that Niblet wouldn't end up as a midnight snack for MooMoo one day. But that didn't stop the fun. The girls would often put Niblet on the dog's head so he could take a ride around the house and you know what? MooMoo didn't seem to mind at all. There seemed to be no end to the fun they could, and did, have with Niblet.

But Niblet was in a quandary. He knew he could help the kids with Wesa's problem, but he rarely got the chance to get near the computer anymore. He needed to study the books Dad had recommended. Together with all of the stuff he learned in the lab with Professor B, he knew he could help Wesa. Occasionally, the kids would take him from the cage and let him run around on the desk while they played or did homework on the computer, but he needed time on his own so that he could work on Wesa's problem. But even more critical, he needed to figure out a way to communicate what he had learned to the kids.

So Niblet hatched a plan, and as difficult as it was going to be for everyone he knew he must go through with it. The idea was this. He had to escape one day so that he could get access to the computer. He would hide in the cupboard way back behind the pans. He knew the perfect spot. Then, when everyone had gone to sleep, he would sneak into the office and go to work. He was going to read all of the books that Dad recommended and he was going to figure out a way of communicating.

Niblet knew that he might have to stay hidden or "lost" for days or perhaps weeks to pull this off, but he couldn't think of another way. It simply wouldn't be good enough to study hard only to have all of the information locked in his head. Nope, he had to find a way to talk with the girls and he knew he needed a computer to do it.

So that was it. It was decided. Niblet would slip away in the afternoon when the girls got home from school and let him out of his cage. He knew they would be sad, but after all, their hamster had gotten away and stayed missing for two whole weeks and showed up again, so he knew that they would not give up hope. And all the while he would be working on this problem…night after night until it was solved.

Around 3:30 that afternoon he heard the garage door open and the sound of the children running into the house. Thump, bump, bam, up the stairs they bounded into their room to get Niblet. They were going to build a grand house for him today out of blocks, and he was going to be the prince of the ball. They had even made some costumes for him to wear and borrowed a hat and glasses from one of their little animal toys. The girls thought he was going to look great. Olivia opened the cage and took Niblet out and put her on the table next to her bed. But, just then she heard her Mom shout, "Olivia, come down here right now and get your backpack and your sweatshirt out of my car. I just had it cleaned."

"Ok, Mom!" shouted back Olivia impatiently. She burst out of the door, slid down the banister, and ran through the garage to get her things from the car. She grabbed her backpack and put it by the door and hung her sweatshirt up on the hook. Off she dashed, up the stairs, back to her room.

Olivia had left Niblet on the table as she often had. But this time it was different. Niblet had seized the opportunity and slipped quietly, quickly, out of the room, down the stairs, into the kitchen and into the cabinet where all of the pans were stored. There was a big pot on the bottom shelf that often blocked the door from closing. He was in luck. The door was open just a bit. Niblet squeezed through the opening and crept behind the old Fondue pot.

And then the whole world sounded as if it were coming to an end. "Mommy!" shouted Olivia. "Niblet is gone. He's gone! I looked under the bed and in the closet and everywhere in my room," she cried nervously. "It's all my fault, I shouldn't have left her out and now she is gone forever."

"No, no it will be all right," her Mom replied. "When Dad gets home he will help you find him."

"But Dad is away for business and he won't be home for days," Olivia cried desperately.

"What will Niblet eat? And what if he ends up in one of the neighbor's mouse traps?" pleaded Olivia.

"Well, you can leave some food out for him, and I'll tell the neighbor to take all of his mousetraps down. Remember, Olivia, Winter was gone for weeks and she came back. Don't you worry, Niblet will come back."

"I guess you're right." said Olivia sadly, as she padded glumly toward the kitchen to get some cups to put out food and water for Niblet. Niblet could hear her coming but he didn't dare show even a little whisker. He needed to stay hidden so that he could solve his own problem and to help Wesa. "Thank heavens she was going to put food out. At least he wouldn't starve to death," thought Niblet.

Niblet was a bit sad for Olivia, but most of all he was excited! He couldn't believe he had actually escaped and hidden himself, but now it was done. Despite his excitement Niblet knew he needed some rest, since he planned to work through the night. So, he curled up behind the old fondue pot and went to sleep.

When he awoke the house was quiet. He could hear Moo-Moo snoring in Giuliana's room as he crept out of the cabinet and into the office. "Now," he thought, "let's hope the computer is still on." He might have to wait another whole night if it wasn't on, because he wasn't sure he could reach the on/off switch. To his delight, he could hear the fan humming on the machine. It was on.

Niblet climbed up the chair and shimmied onto the keyboard tray and then gazed over to the right. "Imposter," he thought as he gazed at the computer mouse. Niblet giggled a bit thinking how Giuliana always loved that joke. But once at the computer, he began to work. He would start by reading the books that Dad had suggested and then brush up on all of the crazy synthetic additives and preservatives he had learned about at the Company. He accessed the online library at the University using Professor B's passwords like he used to do back at the Company. He was able to find most of the books, so he started reading.

Day after day Niblet stayed hidden until he had read all of the books on Dad's list and a whole bunch more. He studied up on the additives even though it made him remember the horrible experiments that his brothers and sisters had taken part in. But, one thing still troubled him. "How was he going to speak with the girls and Wesa?" Niblet kept thinking.

Then one fine night, buried deep in his studies, it came to him. He remembered reading a book about the origins of the universe. Professor B had presented it to him during his studies. Niblet tried hard to remember. "Oh yes, I got it! The book is called, A Brief History of Time by Stephen Hawking." The reason he remembered this so well was that Mr. Hawking was in a wheel chair and could not move almost any part of his body, including his mouth, but he managed to lecture and write books and become world famous in the process. "How did he do it?" thought Niblet. "If a man who can't move a muscle in his body can speak, then so can I," he resolved firmly. So, he began to search the internet and in short order, there it was, in black and white, written by the man himself.

> " I run a program called Equalizer™, written by a company called Words Plus Inc. A cursor moves across the upper part of the screen...In this way I can select words, which are printed on the lower part of the screen. When I have built up a sentence, I can send it to a speech synthesizer. I use a separate synthesizer, made by Speech+...I can also write text using similar menu's to those in Equalizer."

"Wow," thought Niblet, "all I need is the two software packages and the computer will do the rest. This is AWESOME. Houston, we have lift off." he chuckled. Professor B must have known about such software. Maybe he hadn't tried it yet because he wasn't sure that Niblet had learned enough. Now was the time.

He had no doubts about how, nor where, to get what he needed. Professor B had ordered many things as he sat by and watched and he knew the routine well. He went online and found the software, and using Professor B's account, he ordered it to be delivered the next day. He was certain when all was said and done that Professor B would excuse a little dent in his wallet for the satisfaction of knowing that he had succeeded in his crazy pursuit of teaching one little mouse how to read. Of course, now we know, it was much bigger than just that.

The last thing Niblet had to figure out was how to get the kids to load the software when it arrived…and then let him use it. "Ok, I got it." he thought. "I will send a message pretending the software is a present from Professor B. I can send the message from Professor B's which tells them to let ME run around on the keyboard after it is installed, promising a wonderful surprise if they do. Since the email comes from their grandpa, they will surely comply."

Niblet realized the girls might be sad when they saw the software and read the message. It would remind the girls of his absence and could definitely upset them. But Niblet thought of a solution. What he would do was to appear right next to the computer when they got the software, as if it were a grand coincidence. He would hop up on the keyboard and literally blow their ears off.

It was set. If all went according to plan, Niblet would have a way to communicate with the girls and they could move forward working on Wesa's problems. He had read the material that Dad had recommended and he had reviewed all of the crazy studies from the Company that his relatives had endured. "Those were some painful memories. Thank goodness Professor B saved me from all of that." he reflected with mixed emotions.

Niblet knew they would need some good ole' fashion detective work to solve this little "mystery." He determined that once he was "speaking" with the girls he would suggest that they needed to get a peak into Wesa's pantry and figure out just what he was eating. They could take a picture of each label, and bring them home to decipher them. They could compile a list of all of the worst ingredients and anything else that should not be listed in the ingredients declaration. Then, Niblet could explain the potential side effects and harmful aspects of each ingredient. With this information he would suggest creating a "label decoder" which the children could carry around with them and give to their friends. That way they truly could make a difference.

As the night was turning to early morning, Niblet concluded that instead of going to sleep behind the old fondue pot tomorrow, he would sneak into Giuliana's room and hide behind the computer. She was always a little slow in the morning so he could slip in unnoticed and sleep there instead of in the cabinet. That way, right after the kids got the software he could suddenly appear as if by magic. Then he would tell his BIG secret (of course just being able to tell it at all actually is the secret), and he would lay out the big plan. They were going to save Wesa.

6 MISSION TO THE PANTRY

The next morning, as planned, Niblet snuck into Giuliana's room while she was still clearing the fog from her head. He slipped behind her desk and went to sleep. By the time she got back from school he would be well rested and ready to put on his show.

And, that is just the way it happened. Giuliana and Olivia came home from school and found two packages at the door with their names on them. In a mad frenzy of flying paper and shredded cardboard, they opened the boxes. "Software??" They both mumbled quizzically. It wasn't clear to them what the software was for, but it was addressed to them so they decided to load it on their computer. Maybe it was some new game or maybe it was a mistake. Giuliana sat down at her computer, opened her email, and saw a strange message from Professor B.

"It is from Professor B. He wants us to load this software and then see if Niblet will use it. I guess he still thinks that there is something very special about that little mouse. But this email is a little weird. Maybe he's been hacked or something, because this email doesn't look like his writing style at all." said Giuliana. She had been studying such things in her spare time.

"Yeah, right. Maybe it was written by the talking mouse," exclaimed Olivia jovially, twirling her finger around her ear to insinuate the craziness of it all.

"It doesn't matter. Niblet is gone! So there is nothing to do or say. Didn't Grandpa know that Niblet is missing? Why would he send this message to us?" Giuliana snapped. She looked up from the computer and gazed sadly out the window.

"We didn't tell Professor B that we lost Niblet but I was sure that mom and dad did. That must be why he sent this message. He thinks we still have the mouse," she said to Olivia.

"Perhaps but Niblet is going to come back, I just know it." Olivia said firmly and confidently.

And that was his cue, and he wasn't going to miss it. Out from hiding he came.

"NIBLET!" The girls shouted in unison.

Niblet stared back at them smiling. He puffed out his chest and braced himself for the onslaught.

Both girls grabbed for Niblet at the same time, causing him to leap back and onto the computer keyboard, reminding all of them of the new software and the "surprise" that Professor B's message had promised.

"Let's do it right now. Let's get that software installed. I want to know the surprise," Giuliana rattled off quickly.

"Yeah, I wonder what it could be?" shouted Olivia.

"Quiet, calm down. Let's just chillax and do this properly so we don't mess it up," Giuliana implored.

So they loaded the software carefully and completely, and when it was done they put Niblet on the keyboard. With a distinct twinkle in his eye, Niblet browsed through the menus, created a sentence and sent it off to the voice synthesizer

"Hi Girls, my name is Niblet. I have been waiting for this moment for a long time."

"Whatttttttttt is going on?" said Olivia. "Is Niblet talking through the computer?"

"I think so," responded Giuliana in disbelief.

"Yes, it is me, Niblet," the computer voiced.

"Your grandfather taught me to read but I was afraid to communicate after the debacle with the email I sent and all of the problems it caused Professor B. When I saw what happened with Wesa I decided that I must help. I had to find a solution to the communication barrier, and this is it."

"How can you help with Wesa?" Giuliana asked.

"That is a good question" said Niblet. "Let me explain."

"I was born and raised in a lab at a large food company. Professor B kept me out of the food testing studies, but all of my family was in those experiments and I saw the results. Many of the additives that Wesa is sure to be eating were tested there. The other stuff I have been learning about recently during my little sabbatical."

"What do you mean learning about them recently, and what the heck is a sabbatical?" clamored Giuliana.

"Oh, a sabbatical is technically a break that scholars take from their teaching work, often to study something intensively or to write. Anyway, I was listening to the conversation you were having with Dad about Wesa, and I decided to help you so I cooked up the plan to sneak away so that I could spend the nights studying. Once I had completed the books that Dad had recommended, I set out to figure out how to talk to you guys so that I could help," answered Niblet.

"Well how are you going to help? What are we going to do?" Olivia piped in.

Niblet was working the arrow keys like a ten year old on a Nintendo and making sentences as quickly as the synthesizer could push them out. "We are going to use our powers of observation, otherwise known as detective skills. And we are going to find labels from all of the foods that Wesa has been eating. Then we will be able to find out exactly which chemical additives he has actually been consuming. Based on his condition and symptoms, I suspect that he has been eating ingredients that contribute to weight gain and others that are neurotoxins," responded Niblet.

"Neuro-what" asked Olivia.

"Dah, Neurotoxins. Those are things that are poisonous to your brain, right Niblet?" remarked Giuliana.

"That is absolutely correct," confirmed Niblet.

"Wait a minute. Why do people put brain-poison in things that are supposed to be food? I wouldn't even do that and I am only 8," asked Olivia.

"To make them Artificially Delicious, of course," Giuliana quipped.

"Even worse, it appears as though many of the ingredients that are used to artificially enhance flavor and color actually become addictive. That is a boon for the manufacturers, because it keeps people buying more and more of them, but it is harmful for the consumer who is eating too much of a bad thing," explained Niblet.

"What does addictive, mean. It doesn't sound too good?" asked Olivia.

"That is when the body comes to physically need a substance or the person will experience withdrawal symptoms. The person will literally get very sick before they get better if they stop eating the substance," said Niblet.

"Wow! So if Wesa is eating these things, he could have

become addicted to all those chemicals and that is what is causing his ailments. That just sounds wrong on so many levels," pondered Giuliana.

"Yes, that is right. In fact, there are so many harmful and addictive chemicals in the food supply today that it is very hard to avoid them, which is why each person must read the ingredients statement to know what they are eating as we have said." said Niblet.

"So we are going to read all of the labels at Wesa's house?" asked Giuliana. "Sounds like a cool adventure. How are we going to do it?"

"Well, we are going to find a way into Wesa's pantry and you are going to take pictures with your camera so that we can bring them back to the house here and go through the labels one at a time. Then we are going to create the 'Decoder Book' that your friends can use to determine if they are consuming harmful additives and that explains what those additives can do to you," Niblet continued.

"That will be fun," said Olivia. "I can draw a picture for the cover, maybe like a skull and crossbones or something else creepy so the kids will all know that if they see those ingredients on the food then it is bad for them."

"Good idea Olivia," Niblet said approvingly.

"So that is our mission, Olivia," declared Giuliana. "We've gotta go to Wesa's house and get all of the labels from his pantry.

When we bring them back, Niblet can start on the "Decoder Book."

Giuliana called Wesa to find out when they could get into his pantry and refrigerator and decided to set up a play date for the coming Saturday. Wesa's house was very big so they could easily slip in and out of the kitchen without the parents finding out. Giuliana didn't want the parents to get mad about it, so she thought of an excuse.

"It is science, isn't it Olivia?" asked Giuliana

"What do you mean, science? We are talking about decoding the food labels in Wesa's cupboards aren't we?" noted Olivia

"Yeah, but all of those chemicals and stuff are very complicated and technical and require science to produce." said Giuliana

"I guess." Sighed Olivia.

"Well, what I mean is, if they catch us we can just tell them it is a science project so they won't be mad at us for spying on their eating habits," said Giuliana.

"Well, ok. But science and food are not the same thing. Can you picture Grandma cooking up her food in Grandpa's lab, huh? Can you?" said Olivia.

"Well first off, her food doesn't need to last a year on a shelf, so she doesn't not need advanced science. Cooking actually is very much like chemistry in the way that ingredients create reactions in one another and form new compounds. But…and let me say that again…But…that does not mean that we want the actual chemicals from the Lab in our foods," assured Giuliana

"Good Point," said Olivia. "We want FOODS in our FOODS."

So later that week as Saturday came closer the girls readied themselves for their big adventure. I guess you can't really call a play date a big adventure, but the fact is that what they had planned with Niblet was very important to Wesa and it was going to be fun, if perhaps a bit nerve wracking. This was just like one of those Sherlock Holmes books Giuliana loved to read so much. They were going to gather the evidence and then work with Niblet to see if the food could be his problem and, of course, his solution in the end.

Finally Saturday came and the girls left the house around 12:30 with their mother. "What do you want for dinner when you get home," inquired Dad, as they were on their way out the door.

"I don't know," said Olivia

"Doesn't matter," replied Giuliana.

"Well actually, sooner or later you are going to find out that it really does matter." declared Dad.

"Yeah, I know, especially considering what Wesa is going through." said Giuliana.

"This is going to be so cool." exclaimed Olivia as they drove away.

When they arrived at Wesa's house he didn't look very good. If it were possible, he seemed to have gotten worse since they last saw him.

"I feel worse," complained Wesa when the girls asked him how he was.

"I have been getting headaches and all kinds of other weird symptoms. I did go to the Doctor again but they couldn't find anything wrong," Wesa stammered sadly.

"Well we better get right to this little detective job of ours," demanded Olivia. "It looks like Wesa really needs something to pull him out of this health slump he is in."

"Ok, Olivia, you are going to keep watch. Wesa and I will go into the kitchen and start collecting the labels," decided Giuliana.

"If my parents come, just start counting on the wall as if we were playing hide and seek." schemed Wesa.

"We were going to tell them that it was a science project for class," Olivia exclaimed smartly.

So Olivia planted herself at the door at the end of the kitchen leading to the living room. Giuliana and Wesa ventured into the pantry.

"Oh my!" exclaimed Giuliana. "This is bloody outrageous. These are some colorful boxes, huh Wesa? Check out all of the health claims on every package. It is as if eating this things turns you into a super-hero. NOT. This is unbelievable…really."

"This one says, "0g Transfat" "Cholesterol Free" "Good Source of 7 Vitamins and Minerals" and "Good Source of 4 B Vitamins" ; let's look at the ingredients in this product, because it sounds like it must be very healthy," Giuliana continued.

Giuliana took a quick look at the ingredients, and it did not look healthy at all.

ENRICHED FLOUR (WHEAT FLOUR, NIACIN, REDUCED IRON, THIAMIN MONONITRATE [VITAMIN B1], RIBOFLAVIN [VITAMIN B2], FOLIC ACID), CORN SYRUP, HIGH FRUCTOSE CORN SYRUP, DEXTROSE, SOYBEAN AND PALM OIL (WITH TBHQ FOR FRESHNESS), SUGAR, CRACKER MEAL, WHEAT STARCH, SALT, DRIED BLUEBERRIES, DRIED GRAPES, DRIED APPLES, CORNSTARCH, LEAVENING (BAKING SODA, SODIUM ACID PYROPHOSPHATE, MONOCALCIUM PHOSPHATE), CITRIC ACID, CORN CEREAL, GELATIN, PARTIALLY HYDROGENATED SOYBEAN OIL†, MODIFIED CORN STARCH, NATURAL AND ARTIFICIAL BLUEBERRY FLAVOR, MODIFIED WHEAT STARCH, SOY LECITHIN, TRICALCIUM PHOSPHATE, XANTHAN GUM, CARAMEL COLOR, COLOR ADDED, NATURAL AND ARTIFICIAL FLAVOR, TURMERIC EXTRACT, RED #40, VITAMIN A PALMITATE, NIACINAMIDE, REDUCED

IRON, BLUE #2, BLUE #1, PYRIDOXINE HYDROCHLORIDE (VITAMIN B6), RIBOFLAVIN (VITAMIN B2), THIAMIN HYDROCHLORIDE (VITAMIN B1), FOLIC ACID. †LESS THAN 0.5g TRANS FAT PER SERVING

"Wesa, I don't know as much as Niblet, but I always look at the very end of the ingredient label because we are not allowed to eat artificial colors or flavors, and they always put those at the end of the label. It looks like there is more than one artificial color in this product."

"Wow" Said Wesa, "Are you sure those aren't all of the colors they used on the snappy box that these came in?" Wesa chuckled.

"Yes, I am sure Wesa. By the way, this is not funny at all. Look at the label, and see how long the ingredient list is. That is almost always a bad sign and a quick indicator to find another food option. Now, look at the end of the list to see if they have used artificial colors or flavors. They always list those near the end of the list, so it can save you the time of reading through all of the other ingredients. Colors with numbers have no place in your food because they are made from Petroleum and they have been definitively linked to the problems with focus and concentration that you have been experiencing. Dad told me there are many studies which have concluded that simply eliminating artificial colors from one's diet improves behavior and test scores in children. Since you have been having concentration problems, artificial colors should be the first thing you stop eating," Giuliana said firmly.

Just then Olivia started counting very slowly and very loudly. "One, two, three…"

And as she did, Wesa and Giuliana froze in the Pantry. They stared at each other in the partial light coming in from the crack in the slightly open door.

They heard Olivia counting but no other voices were audible. Olivia finished counting to ten. "Ready or not, here I come." She shouted as she started walking toward the pantry to peak in.

Now, they could all hear the sound of light footsteps and thought for certain that they were going to be caught. Wesa was on a diet and wasn't supposed to be in the pantry at all between meals.

"Tell them that it's a science project, remember, because it really is," whispered Giuliana.

"Ok," Wesa responded quietly.

And just as the steps started to reach the door they realized what it was.

"It's just the DOG," said Olivia as Wesa's dog came around the corner panting and wagging.

"Who's a good girl?" Olivia said as she gave the dog a hug.

"Whew, that was scary. Let's get these pictures of the

labels quickly so we can go home. I'm sure this insane collection of colorful boxes is your problem. There is no doubt. I remember a lot of those things from my Uncle's pantry. Dad took us through there one day just for fun to see how crazy an ingredient label can really be. With these pictures and Niblet's help, we are going to figure out exactly what is going on here," Giuliana said smartly.

Giuliana and Wesa worked quickly. He grabbed the boxes and she shot pictures of the ingredient declaration on each of the many boxes in the pantry. The cereal, the stuffing mix, the gravy, and so on and so forth. Then they tackled the freezer, going through it quickly and shooting the pictures. Just as they were finishing up Wesa's mom came in to the kitchen from the sliding glass door that led to the pool.

"Hey kids, how are you? You must be very hungry. Olivia and Giuliana, your mother asked me to give you lunch if you want it." Wesa's Mom said.

"No, no, that is ok. We are not hungry right now. You know what Dad always says, "eat when you are hungry and drink when you are thirsty,"" Giuliana said, winking at Olivia. She definitely did not want to eat any of those things in that pantry even if they were tempting.

"ARTIFICIALLY DELICIOUS, ARTIFICIALLY DELICIOUS, ARTIFICIALLY DELICIOUS," Olivia reminded herself over and over.

"Well, that's ok with me. You kids just let me know when you are hungry," Wesa's mom said.

But the girls never did admit to being hungry that afternoon, and when Dad came to pick them up they were famished.

"Why didn't you eat something at Wesa's house?" asked Dad as the kids pleaded for him to stop for food.

"Dad, you really can't imagine all of the crazy things we found in Wesa's kitchen. I did not find one thing that you would have approved of so we just told his mom we weren't hungry," said Giuliana.

"I'm bringing a bag of snacks and stuff next time. I love to play at his house but we need to figure out the food situation," said Olivia. She was a voracious eater and could hardly be without food for any period of time much less a whole afternoon.

"Dad, did you know that Wesa and Giuliana copied every label in the kitchen?" said Olivia, spilling the proverbial beans.

"No, I did not. Does this have something to do with the things we talked about earlier and trying to figure out what his health issues are?" Dad inquired.

"Yes, but it is much deeper than that," responded Giuliana mysteriously.

"What do you mean by 'Much deeper than that' Giu Giu?" said Dad.

"Well, do you remember all of that crazy work that Professor B was doing with Niblet? Trying to educate him and trying to get him to speak?" Giuliana continued.

"Uh, yes, what does that have to do with the price of eggs in China?" quipped Dad.

"Let's just say it worked," said Giuliana.

"What worked?" asked Dad, now piquing his interest.

"All of his work, 'worked'," Giuliana replied coyly.

"Huh? He quit after he couldn't prove that he had succeeded with Niblet. So, why are you telling me now that "it worked"?" Dad groaned.

"Ok, you remember when Niblet disappeared for several weeks?" asked Giuliana.

"Yes Giuliana, he only returned just this week." Dad said shortly.

"Right, well, while he was away, he read all of those books you recommended and he figured out how to talk to us using computer software to synthesize a voice and some other program that allows him to quickly make sentences," Giuliana confessed.

"Yeah, right, and you have also got a bridge in Brooklyn to sell me right, or some nice land in the Arizona desert?" said Dad

"Dad, I am telling you the truth. Niblet can talk now and he knows all about the ingredients in the foods. He told us that he had been briefed on all of the relevant food additive studies during his time in the lab with Professor B. And he is the one that told us to sneak around and get labels from Wesa's kitchen," Giuliana implored.

"Sneak around?" Dad said.

"Well we didn't exactly want to be gawking at all of that stuff in their house that they think is food, and Wesa is not supposed to go into the cupboards or pantry because he's on a strict diet. So we sort of made it into a scientific detective game and we gathered evidence. Now we are going to take the ingredient listings to Niblet and De-Code them together. And then we are going to make a "Super Label Detective Decoder Book" that we can give to all of the kids to help them as well." she said.

"Now that sounds like a very interesting, albeit completely unbelievable, story," said Dad. "You have got yourself a doozy there. You should write that down some day."

"It's truuuuuuuuuue Daaaaaaaaaad. You'll see," said Olivia firmly.

Something about the way Olivia said that opened a window of possibility in Dad's mind about the validity of the story they had told. True or not, she certainly believed it.

And after all, whether or not Niblet could speak, the Decoder book was a good idea. Dad decided he was going to be sure that they got it done because Wesa wasn't the only child around who needed guidance in choosing foods. If they could teach the children, maybe the children would teach the parents.

That night Giuliana texted Wesa.

"I tld dad abt the thng wr dng. He sd he wld hlp. Gd Nt, W. Yr gonna feel btr soon." She wrote.

"Thnx. Gd nyt, I realy hope so. Ur nvr guna beat me again!" he replied.

And as Giuliana laid her head down on her pillow to sleep that night she began to think about Wesa's problem.

Giuliana remembered a famous study that was conducted in New York City Schools in the 70's and early 80's that Dad always talked about. They changed the foods to avoid chemical additives, especially dyes, and their test scores went up dramatically over the next couple of years, well beyond any gains in previous years. That would certainly help any school, especially now that funding was based on performance.

For some crazy reason they stopped doing it. But, at least the study showed how effective a good diet can be on improving learning. Dad said that there were are lot of other schools that had made similar changes to their food and experienced better behavior, as well as higher test scores.

This is complicated she thought. If there is so much evidence that we perform better without these chemicals and additives, why can't we just leave them out? Oh yeah, she remembered, the "FOODS" need to look and taste the same after a whole year on the shelf so a lot of food science is required, like Michael Pollan always talks about. Creeeeepy!

As she slowly faded off to sleep Giuliana began to dream. In her dream Wesa was strong and healthy and was graduating at the top of his class. His parents were alongside him and they looked surprisingly spry as well. Her dream moved to the garden next to the cafeteria at the school where people from the community came every week to help care for the produce. She could sense deep down that Niblet was responsible! What a mouse.

7 IDENTIFYING THE WORST INGREDIENTS

All through the next week Giuliana was thinking about the project with Wesa. She was going to meet him on Saturday to go over the labels with Niblet. She was trying to figure out the best way to go about it. There were so many different substances in the foods in Wesa's cupboard that they could not possibly decode all of them.

"We had better devise a strategy Niblet." Giuliana said.

"Don't worry Giuliana. We are going to start with the ingredients that are artificial. You know, things that did not start out as food, but as something else. What you will find is every one of these ingredients had been physically or chemically altered, even supposed 'Natural' ingredients. After that we will learn how to read the label, including the nutrient panel," Niblet replied. "If we tried to comprehend every chemical in today's so-called foods, we would be overwhelmed. So, we will focus on the most commonly used problem additives. Avoiding those will go a long way to restoring your health."

When Saturday arrived, Wesa's mom brought him over to the Girls' house for a "play date" or to "hang out" as Giuliana liked to say. She could hardly appreciate or know the importance of the work they would be doing that day.

Wesa was a touch apprehensive because he wasn't sure he would understand everything Niblet was going to tell them. But he was sure that Giuliana would help, and besides, he had to find a solution to his problem. He most definitely did not want to take those pills the Doctor had prescribed, and his mom said if his situation did not improve she would force him to take them.

They all gathered in Giuliana's room and Niblet stood on her desk next to the computer, ready to begin the lecture. The kids still couldn't believe they were about to be schooled on nutrition by a mouse, but hey, it was also pretty cool. If he could help save Wesa, they were all ears!

"Uh, so where should we start," asked Wesa.

Niblet jumped up on the touch-pad on the laptop and started grooving around it like he was ice-skating; lining up sentences and sending them to the voice synthesizer one after another. It was sort of funny that a little mouse's slipping and sliding would change these children's lives forever. But that is how it was.

"Well, let's begin by saying there are literally thousands of individual chemicals in the foods and most have not had adequate long term studies conducted on them," the artificial voice that would be Niblet began. "Some are used to sweeten, others to color, others to preserve, moisten, soften, and what have you. In traditional foods, this was done with natural ingredients, the most basic being salt and sugar. Both of these enhance flavor and also preserve. In moderation, they have been proven safe for millennia. What you need to grasp, is the fact that every problem ingredient is artificial or has been physically or chemically altered from its natural state," said Niblet.

"But not all chemicals and additives are bad, are they Niblet?" asked Wesa.

"No Wesa, in fact our bodies, our food, everything is comprised of chemicals. However, some chemicals, both natural and man-made can affect our bodies adversely and thus should be not be ingested. These are things that nature did not intend us to eat," said Niblet.

"So, where do we begin?" Wesa asked coyly.

"Let's start with ingredients that other countries have already banned or restricted, based on their scientific discoveries, given that our oversight agencies are not overzealous about restricting additives from our food supply. For instance, the European Union has far stricter standards than we do on food additives. When there is doubt about the safety of a food product or additive, it is removed from the system until it has been proven safe," said Niblet.

"The Precautionary Principle!" Giuliana barked.

"You got it!" said Niblet.

"What is the Precautionary Principle?" asked Olivia.

"Yes, I too am Curious," Wesa cut in.

"The Precautionary Principle in science states that if you can't prove something is safe, you don't use it. Isn't that right Niblet?" Giuliana asked; all the while knowing she was right.

"Right again. Yet what prevails in our country today is the opposite. What I mean is, in the USA if something hasn't been proven beyond-doubt to be absolutely deadly, then we use it. And, magically, every single time a study shows that any specific ingredient MAY be problematic, industry churns out a study showing the opposite, and thus we continue with our upside down view of the Precautionary Principle."

"Wait, that is too much information," said Wesa. "What does that really mean?"

"It simply means that we have to educate ourselves, weigh the evidence, and make good choices for ourselves. The system is not going to protect us the way we think it should," Niblet responded.

"Well, that IS why we are here Niblet. To edumacate ourselves about these here nasty additives thingeees," chirped Olivia. "So…let's do it!"

"I love your enthusiasm! To begin, there are many different types of additives, both synthetic and natural, both good and bad. Some additives are used to preserve things, making them last much longer than nature intended. Others are used to create flavors or colors for which nature has no equal or which are addicting to the consumer. And of course there are sweeteners, and softeners and conditioners, stabilizers, and on and on and on. There are literally thousands of chemicals entering the food every year with little or no oversight," said Niblet.

"I just can't to believe this is true." Wesa said anxiously.

"It is true Wesa. Trust me. What's the first category Niblet? We need to get started." Giuliana stated solemnly.

Artificial Colors: Petrolium Dyes, Colors with Numbers

"Let's begin with artificial colors and dyes, because they affect the most important part of our body, your brain. Recent studies done in England suggested that artificial colors and dyes can play a significant role in Attention Deficit Disorder and ADHD? In one study, children taking drugs for these disorders were asked to eliminate colors from their diets and the result was almost two thirds didn't need medication any longer. Medications like the ones your doctor recommended Wesa. As a result of these studies, the three major supermarket chains removed all of these artificial colors and dyes from their store shelves. Now that makes a lot of sense," said Niblet.

"Studies about artificial colors and petroleum dyes have also been done here Niblet," Giuliana interjected. "In fact the Feingold Program has been investigating and advocating for removal of these artificial dyes since the 70's. Dad always talks about schools that have improved test scores and behavior simply by removing this one ingredient. Dyes are derived from petroleum, so it is no wonder they removed them from the store shelves in England. The manufacturers simply switched to non-synthetic colors and the products still look and taste just the same as they did before."

"So, if they have removed the artificial dyes but are still selling the same types of products, they proved that we do not need them, right Niblet," said Wesa.

"Exactly, Wesa. Not only are they toxic, they are superfluous," replied Niblet.

"Toxic Superfoods? Awesome. That's good right?" Olivia jumped in.

"No Olivia, toxic means deadly, like your dirty socks. And superfluous means, NEEDLESS or UNNECESSARY. We don't need to make things in colors which have no equeal in nature, especially if they are toxic!" said Giuliana.

"So, artificial colors will be the first thing we list as problematic because we should not be eating things derived from crude oil. They have been shown to be problematic, and they are superfluous," Said Niblet.

"Yes, sir, my little tiny professor, got it." So she typed into her laptop 'Artificial Colors'. "Got it. What is next?" chirped Giuliana.

Artificial Preservatives:

BHA, BHT, TBHQ, Sodium Benzoate, Sodium Nitrate, Sodium Nitrite

"Let's talk about preservatives. Believe it or not, there are many preservatives in use today that have been banned in other countries for decades. Three of the worst culprits are normally listed by their initials instead of their long scary scientific names. They appear as BHA, BHT and their modern cousin TBHQ, and don't sound nearly as nefarious as they are. All three of these affect behavior as well, as has been documented scientifically. And while we are at it, we should also list Sodium Benzoate, Sodium Nitrate and Sodium Nitrite which many recent studies have indicated to be extremely problematic," said Niblet.

"What are preservatives used for?" said Olivia.

"Dah, to "preserve" things," Giuliana jumped in, as if that answered it for Olivia.

"Well they make things last a long time, but unfortunately they can be harmful to your health, and in large quantities they can even be fatal. I remember one of the studies we conducted with Professor B on TBHQ which proved that just five grams of the TBHQ can be fatal to a human being," said Niblet.

"WHAAAAA! Fatal, that means deadly, right?" cried Wesa. "One of the labels in my Pantry said, "Canola or Palm oil with TBHQ for Freshness". That implies that this is something good and something that I would actually want."

"Of course it does. It sounds better than "with TBHQ to

make sure this thing doesn't spoil for the next two years on the shelf at the big box store supply chain," joked Niblet. "It's all done with words, and they are often misleading."

"But it's not 'Fresh', it just sort of looks that way, right Niblet?" said Giuliana.

"You tell me," replied Niblet.

"Wait, wait, wait. You are saying that if the machine in the factory is calibrated incorrectly and dispenses too much TBHQ my candy wrapper then I could actually DIE from this?" Wesa asked.

"In large quantities it can be fatal, so the FDA restricts its usage to very small amounts. The real problem is that even in very small concentrations it has been definitively shown to effect behavior, as I said. And unfortunately it is everywhere; from the wrappers on Wheat Crackers to Chewing Gum to Chicken Nuggets, so people are ingesting far more of it that they realize," said Niblet.

"I recently reviewed a copy of Eater's Digest written over 40 years ago. It says quite clearly that BHA and BHT have no place in our food due to their poisonous nature. TBHQ was not yet in common use. That fact that they still have not removed these substances is clearly a matter of politics and not good sense," Niblet continued. "But, that same book gave a clean bill of health for Sodium Benzoate which is widely used in soft drinks and dark colored sauces to preserve them. Recent studies have definitively shown that Sodium Benzoate can break down into the known carcinogen, benzene. If that were not bad enough, other studies have indicated that it can disrupt the mitochondria of the DNA, actually damaging the cells."

"So, even if some additives appear ok today, we may discover their problematic nature later. That is why it is always best to avoid them whenever possible, right?" quizzed Wesa.

"You got it Wesa. Eat foods!" Olivia replied smartly.

"Niblet, you are going too fast. I know that a carcinogen is something that causes cancer, but what on God's green earth is a mitochondria?" Giuliana asked.

"Correct, a Carcinogen is something that causes cancer." replied Niblet. "Mitochondria are the structures in certain cells that create usable energy from what we eat."

"Your are saying that Sodium Benzoate is carcinogenic AND can damage the exact part of the body that gets energy from food? That's not exactly what I would want in a food additive," said Wesa. "Niblet, what is it actually doing to the Mitochondria?"

"Well that is very complicated, but let's just suffice it to say that your body is being damaged on a cellular level," said Niblet.

"Niblet, how could anyone put these harmful additives in the food?" Wesa asked desperately.

"They do so because they can. Nobody is demanding better. As with the case of the artificial colors in England, if the consumer demands better, industry will deliver. Most people are not aware of what they are eating, and they don't really care to be.

If we all learn to make better choices and demand cleaner products, industry will respond as they have in Great Britain, and so many other places," Niblet lectured.

"Wow. Simply eating the wrong things can damage our health; right down to the building blocks of our cells. So, I will write down the Artificial Preservatives, BHT, BHA and TBHQ and also Sodium Benzoate. We will label them as preservatives. What are they made from?" Giuliana asked.

"BHA, BHT and TBHQ are made from Petroleum, but Sodium Benzoate is not. But, interesting tidbit, sodium benzoate can be used effectively as an ingredient in home-made rocket fuel!" Niblet revealed.

"Rocket fuel? Great!" squealed Giuliana. "What is it with the crude oil and propellants in our food supply? Isn't it painfully obvious to anyone that Petroleum is not for consumption by people. Niblet, so many of these additives harm our brains, and they seem to be working together to dumb us down!"

"Maybe that was not the intention, but it is the result." Niblet lamented. "Avoiding chemicals that affect our brains may seem obvious, but people consume them because they believe the food supply is safe. In the end, this is about personal responsibility. Each of us must educate ourselves, read the ingredients and make good choices for their personal health," Niblet said sternly, staring directly at Wesa.

"I guess you are right." said Wesa, "But you can't expect everyone to be a scientist. Isn't that what the oversight agencies in the Government are for?"

"Sadly, the letter agencies in Washington have a long history of protecting industry and allowing problem ingredients to enter the food supply. Agency heads often come from the very companies they are supposed to regulate. As a result, companies have even won rulings that allow them to put known problematic additives in the food. Examples are the carcinogenic preservatives Sodium Nitrate and Sodium Nitrite. The World Cancer Research Center has recommended that people avoid processed luncheon meats and hot dogs altogether due to the Nitrates and Nitrites, yet the companies argued that it kills bacteria so the FDA has let it pass despite its carcinogenic nature. But many brands do not contain Nitrates or Nitrites, so clearly they are Superfluous. Right Olivia?" Niblet shot back.

"Superfluous. Not necessary. Got it," said Olivia. "Did you add Sodium Nitrite and Nitrate to the list?"

"I did Olivia. It's a preservative," Giuliana said impatiently.

"Did you just say that additives can be approved for use in the food supply even if there is concrete evidence that they are potentially harmful?" asked Wesa.

"It has happened. In some cases, companies simply keep applying for approval until their pleas fall on sympathetic ears regardless of prior denials," Niblet said. "The motivation for profit has no moral compass."

"Isn't aspartame a good example of this?" Said Giuliana.

Artificial Sweeteners: Aspartame, Acelfame, etc.

"Yes, unfortunately it is. And Artificial Sweeteners should be the next group of ingredients which we include. Some have been shown to be problematic for years, yet they are extremely prevalent," Niblet replied. "There are a whole bunch of them with many different names, and you should avoid them all. The most widely recognized independent scientific advocacy group, Center for Science in the Public Interest has clearly recommended that the most commonly used artificial sweeteners, Aspartame, Acelfame K and Saccharin all be avoided for various health reasons."

"What was that crazy story I read about Aspartame again?" Asked Giuliana.

"That would be far too long to tell right now," said Niblet. "Suffice it to say, the Bressler Report reviewed the manufacturer's science and it borders on criminal. Brain tumors were removed and not reported, rodents were re-incarnated who had died early in the experiment, and many other serious breaches of scientific practice were found. Despite this, the sweetener was approved when one very well connected person took the helm at the corporation producing it. Over the years, the FDA has given it a clean bill of health despite numerous contradictory studies. It is addictive, poisonous and extremely hazardous to your health. And once again it affects the same parts of your brain that help you learn and concentrate," reported Niblet.

"I saw an episode of 60 minutes from 1996, which laid out the pro's and cons of aspartame. The fact is, that of the 166 aspartame studies done up to that point, those that were funded by industry gave a clean bill of health in 100 percent of those studies, while those not funded by industry indicated problems with Aspartame 92 percent of the time. In other words, virtually all independent studies showed problems, and yet it is today considered by the FDA to be one of the most tested and safe additives in the food supply. So you tell me, using the precautionary principle and looking at the evidence, have we proven it's safety?" Niblet asked rhetorically.

Wesa weighed in, "The evidence would suggest that we have not proven it's safety despite all of the propaganda and hype surrounding it."

"One of the weirdest things about these sweeteners is that due to their extremely addictive nature, you now find them in places you would never expect. So, you must read every label, even in your old favorites," said Niblet. "Most people drink artificially sweetened products to avoid the calories that sugar delivers. They believe that eating fewer calories will help with weight problems, and normally it would. However, long term studies on thousands of diet soda drinkers have found that they actually gained weight because these sweeteners make your body crave carbohydrates, causing people to over-eat."

"Your are saying that so-called "DIET" products can actually make you fat?" Cried Wesa. "No wonder my parents have had such a hard time taking off the pounds. My pantry is full of this stuff."

"OK, I put all of those Artificial Sweeteners on the list," Giuliana said softly, clearly a bit overwhelmed by all of this.

"Hey, would it be good to read the label in reverse to see if they contain any Artificial Colors, Artificial Sweeteners or Dangerous preservatives, like Giuliana told me the other day?" asked Wesa.

Artificial and "Natural flavors"

"That works for all of the additives we have already spoken about. Another class of additives listed at the end of the label is flavors, both artificial and "natural." Artificial flavors are used to create taste sensations that are consistent, powerful, addicting and sometime manipulate the senses. The FDA recently approved an "artificial flavor" that acts more like a drug than a food, and there was only a three month safety study done. Now how much could you know about the health risks of an ingredient after only three months? Cigarettes take years and years to cause cancer but nobody is in doubt as to their dangerous nature," declared Niblet.

"Interesting tidbit on Artificial Flavors Niblet!" interrupted Giuliana. "Did you know that Vanillin, the most commonly used artificial vanilla flavoring, is a by-product of highly toxic paper pulp production? Paper mills routinely put a vanillin plant nearby so they can turn their waste into our food additives. Can you say WIEEEERD?"

"WiEEEERD," Olivia mocked.

"That is true Giuliana, in fact many artificial flavors are

similarly concocted from a macabre of industrial chemicals. However, we have to look out for so-called "Natural" Flavors as well," said Niblet.

"Yeah, just because something is "natural" does not mean it is healthy," Giuliana jumped in excitedly. "We have a castor bean plant growing in our backyard which is listed in my world record book as the most poisonous plant on earth, 1600 times more poisonous than rattlesnake venom I believe. And yet, it's 100 percent "natural". Now do you get the idea?"

"Precisely, "natural" means not man-made, it does not mean healthy or problem free. A naturally wholesome food product does not need to be labeled just as "Natural Flavoring." They can further disclose it as "peppermint oil" like your Altoids if there is nothing to hide. Remember, very strange things can be concealed within the term "natural'."

"Well, Dad always says, 'Tires are natural but I wouldn't want to eat one,'" Giuliana joked.

"Yes, tires are made from rubber which "naturally" comes from a tree. But they are not food. Much in the same way, many things that are termed 'natural' can very well be non-foods which is exactly what we are trying to avoid," said Niblet.

"Ok, I am adding Artificial and "Natural" flavors to our list. Right Niblet?" queried Giuliana.

Soy Proteins:

"Yes, but remember not all "natural" flavors are bad, you just have to be wary when they don't explain what the additive is made from," Niblet replied. "While we are on the subject of natural, did you know that most so-called "natural" Veggie Burgers and other plant based, soy proteins are derived using Hexane Gas which is a byproduct of... "You Guessed It" gasoline production. These vegetable proteins are advertised as healthy, 'Natural', and vegetarian, but they contain residues of the gas from production. Independent tests have shown residue levels at twice the amount allowed in Europe where limits are set on these chemicals. Your soy protein is bound to have chemical residues the processing unless it is labeled Organic."

"I need to add Non-Organically processed soy proteins Niblet?" Giuliana clarified.

"Yes. I know the list is getting long, but all the these ingredients are important to look at," replied Niblet.

"How many more things can we focus on?" asked Giuliana.

"Well, the chemicals we have already discussed can be dangerous when used as food additives and almost every one of them has detrimental effects on behavior and learning. Many have also been banned or are no longer in use in other countries. But there is another whole class of foods and additives that seem to be directly contributing to the obesity epidemic. Didn't you say that

Wesa had gained a lot of weight since he was adopted?" asked Niblet.

"Yes, he did gain weight, and I actually beat him in a foot race. He used to be the fastest kid in the orphanage but not so much anymore. Even worse, his studies are not going well. The additives we already discussed could be responsible for that. Sister D always said he was the brightest star in the class," reflected Giuliana sadly.

"Well, if he is eating processed foods then there is a very good chance that he is consuming one or more substances that has been shown to play a role in obesity," said Niblet.

"Which additives are the worst in this regard?" asked Giuliana.

HFCS: High Fructose Corn Syrup

"Let's start with the one that everyone blames," said Niblet. "The rise in obesity directly parallels the introduction and increase in the consumption of High Fructose Corn Syrup in the United States."

"Wait, didn't we see a bunch of T.V. commercials that said HFCS is just the same as sugar?" Giuliana asked.

"That is funny, and it is "natural' too, right?" said Niblet.

"Yes, 'natural,' just like tires," Giuliana quipped.

"There have been many studies regarding the harmful

effects of consuming HFCS. They have shown everything from liver damage to Metabolic Syndrome. Recently an extensive study has linked it to the rise in Type 2 Diabetes. And yet another at Princeton University showed that HFCS has a direct role in obesity. In the experiment, all of the rodents that ate the HFCS got fat and those eating table sugar did not. And the rodents eating the HFCS were getting fewer calories. It was pretty simple," said Niblet.

"What is Metabolic Syndrome? I have heard a lot about that recently," Wesa said puzzled.

"Metabolic Syndrome is a combination of risk factors which can lead to heart disease and diabetes. Some suggest that as many as 25% of Americans suffer from this. A recent UC Davis study showed that indicators of this disease cluster could begin within two short weeks of consuming HFCS," Niblet continued. "Previous research suggested that HFCS actually changes the appetite regulating hormones, so your "I'm Full" mechanism doesn't work properly, causing people to overeat. If that weren't bad enough, we know that many samples of HFCS contain mercury as a result of the method of processing. Mercury is not safe at any level, so although we have been told that HFCS is the same as table sugar in its makeup, there is a huge body of research that suggests otherwise."

"Wow, that was a mouthful, but it seems pretty clear that HFCS is not something I want to eat," Wesa gasped.

"Yes, but the recent media blitz by the Corn Board created

doubt among many consumers, despite all of the research," added Niblet. "And yet, all of the major soda manufacturers and processed food giants have been changing their recipes and are putting prominent "NO HFCS" labels on the packaging. So, if it is not a problem, then what is going on here? The answer of course is that the truth about HFCS is not pretty."

"Ok, so I will write down High Fructose Corn Syrup. What are the other Obesigens that we need to cover?" plied Giuliana.

"You should write down HFCS but remember this: the industry is trying to re-brand the product as Corn Sugar so we may soon have to watch out for that too," continued Niblet.

"I guess their confusion campaign wasn't that successful if they are now changing the name," said Giuliana.

"That is one way to look at it. But the problem is that people are eating way too much of it. Everything from Ketchup to Salad Dressing and even Bread contains HFCS, so watch out kiddo."

"HFCS, Corn Sugar, CHECK," Giuliana mumbled aloud as she typed. "Next?"

Hydrogenated Oils:

"Another problem ingredient that has gotten a lot of attention but is still very present in our food supply is Partially Hydrogenated Oil and the Trans fats it delivers. These have a very bad effect on Cholesterol levels, which can lead to heart problems, one of the leading causes of death in the United States," said Niblet. "They are so bad that the USDA actually changed the labeling requirements to include a trans-fat section."

"Hydro…what oil?" asked Giuliana

"Hydrogenated, Giuliana," responded Niblet. "It means that Hydrogen has been added. This creates a very bad fat from a good one using serious science. It's a really neat trick. You take something that is essentially healthy and modify it in a way that makes it toxic to humans. And then you put it in everything because it has beneficial manufacturing properties despite the fact that we know it to be absolutely terrible for your health."

"Why on Earth would we want to change a good fat into a bad one, and by the way, aren't all fats bad?" Pondered Giuliana.

"No Giuliana, your body and especially your brain need good naturally occurring fats to survive. Although fats have been vilified, the China Study and a body of recent research has shown that the animal proteins, not Fat, are the real culprit. In fact, in the 60's there was a very successful campaign by the sugar industry to vilify dietary cholesterol and fat as the culprit in heart disease and high blood lipid levels, when in fact evidence by many scholars showed that not to be the case. After decades of poisoning the people with Hydrogenated Oils, we now know that they are far worse than the saturated fats that they replaced," detailed Niblet.

"Chemistry plus food equals everlasting, artificially delicious, albeit completely toxic treats. What a system we have going here!" reflected Giuliana.

"Wait, if Hydrogenated Oils have gotten so much attention, why are they still being used?" asked Wesa.

"That is a good question. Everyone is focused on the horrible "Trans-Fats" that Hydrogenated Oil delivers and the label guidelines were even changed to include a "Trans Fat" listing several years ago as I mentioned. So, people now look for "Trans Fats" on the Nutrient Panel and the claims of "Zero Trans Fats" on the packages. BUT, since anything less than 0.5 grams "per serving" is listed as zero, industry just changed the level of hydrogenation and adjusted the serving sizes. Do you see how the game works?" instigated Niblet.

"So, even when the nutrient panel says Zero trans-fats, they could still be in my food?" asked Giuliana. "One serving may contain less than a half gram and thus be called zero, but who eats one serving of anything? And if someone eats the whole box, then they will be eating a lot of "trans fats" despite the "Zero" claim on the package. Is that it Niblet?"

"Yes Giuliana, that is why you have to look for the words Partially Hydrogenated Oil," declared Niblet. "Manufacturers are still using Hydrogenated oils, and in reality, we don't know if the levels of trans fats claimed on the label are actually correct."

"For example, trans fats are so bad that New York City banned them in all of the more than 20,000 restaurants in the city. Unfortunately, even after they claimed to have removed them, independent testing showed significant amounts of trans-fats. The trans-fat situation is worse than ever because now they are hiding behind claims of Zero. So you must carefully read the ingredient declaration," Niblet implored.

"EWWW, scary…Hidden Trans-Fats. It's like a bad horror movie. It is clear that we should definitely avoid Hydrogenated Oils. I am putting on the list." said Giuliana tapping away at her keyboard.

Stripped Enriched Bleached Flours:

"Moving along, let's talk about bleached "enriched" flours and other stripped carbohydrates like white rice," continued Niblet

"Ok," Giuliana responded. "I know about this one. Dad always says that your body treats simple carbohydrates such as "enriched" flour just as though it were sugar. So we always say that you can eat a bagel but think of it like a donut, it is desert unless it is whole grain."

"Recent science is pointing to the glycemic index as a better way to look at foods, where certain foods are intrinsically higher in simple starches than others. But the gist of what you are saying is correct. Complex carbohydrates, otherwise known as whole grains contain more nutrients, fiber, and minerals than their stripped cousins. What else did you learn?" asked Niblet.

"Well, they created the process to grind flour with steel rollers late in the 19th century, but the final product had almost zero nutrients. All of the healthy parts of the wheat grain were removed leaving only the simple carbohydrate. Years later the government forced companies to 'enrich' the flour with B Vitamins and Folic acid to make up for the lost nutrients because the military and the government were concerned that too many of the nations' young people were not fit for service. People were getting diseases only associated with severe malnutrition because they were eating this flour," said Giuliana.

"But that is where it gets "funny," Giuliana said, using her fingers to make quotation marks when she said funny. "I mean, why did they call it enriched if they remove more than 30 nutrients and vitamins and then add back 5?"

Niblet rubbed his brow and took a deep breath. Sometimes this conversation really did make him sad. But Giuliana knew a lot about this, and that made him feel better. Wesa was going to do just fine with friends like her around.

"Yes, we really should be calling it what it really is 'stripped flour', not enriched. Imagine the Sheriff of Nottingham storming the village and taking all of the food as tax. Then feeling a tinge philanthropic, the Sheriff gives back barely enough food for the villagers to survive. Would you consider these people 'enriched', or simply robbed?" asked Niblet.

"Naturally we would have to conclude that they were not enriched," responded Wesa.

"That is exactly the problem with 'Enriched Flour'. Most of the essential vitamins and nutrients which the body vitally needs are removed and then convenient versions of a few B vitamins and folic acid are added back. You must look at the ingredient statement and see the words 'Whole' before the grain to know that you are getting the complete food and not a stripped version."

"Yes, and Dad says if it does not say 'Whole' than it is definitely stripped. Regardless of whether it is wheat, barley, or whatever," added Giuliana.

"Right, and this is one of the tricks that fools so many people," continued Niblet. "People see 'Multi-Grain' or 'Wheat' and think it's healthier, but it is only better if there are 'Whole Grains'. So we have to make sure we read and find the word WHOLE," said Niblet.

"WHOLE grains do not break down in the system like simple carbohydrates, so you don't get the immediate blood sugar rise followed by the crash. They are digested more slowly so the energy is released over time, right?" queried Giuliana

"The fact is, when we eat foods that have very little nutrient value we never feel satisfied because the human body is very sophisticated and knows intrinsically that it needs certain nutrients. When it does not find them in the stripped down food it keeps asking for every greater quantities in the effort to get the nutrients essential for good health. Farmers call this Hay Belly with their cows. The result is that people, and cows for that matter, who eat nutrient-poor food end up being fat because they just keep eating. We now have a whole generation of people that are obese but malnourished. In fact, the Military is once again sounding the alarm that too many of our nations' youth are not fit to serve," said Niblet.

"Now that is just weird. I never thought that someone could be fat and also malnourished. I guess if you don't eat whole foods you will not get the proper nutrients no matter how much you eat," reflected Giuliana.

"In general, kids, you should avoid foods that are making claims such as "lite," "diet," etc. They have removed calories by adding stripped and artificial ingredients but often these foods are absolutely void of nutrients," declared Niblet.

Giuliana looked at Wesa and Olivia. They seemed a bit overwhelmed by Niblet's lecture. "Niblet, are we almost done?" asked Giuliana. "I am not sure how much more of this we can retain today."

MSG and Free Glutamates:

"Well, Kids, I wanted to go over the last major problem ingredient category which is Free Glutamates. Tomorrow we will look at some labels to better understand how to read them and what to look for." responded Niblet.

"What are Free Glutamates and are there slave-glutamates?" Olivia joked.

"Well the best known Free Glutamates is call "MSG" or mono-sodium Glutamate. MSG was associated with a whole range of symptoms from headaches to seizures all the way back in 1968. Reactions to MSG came to be known as Chinese Restaurant Syndrome, as Chinese restaurants used to be the biggest users of MSG, but today you will find them lurking everywhere," said

Niblet.

"Behind the corner, out of sight, and ready to do, "what exactly!" asked Olivia.

"Paaaleeease," Giuliana said sarcastically.

"What is wrong with Glutamates?" asked Wesa.

"In their natural state they do not present a problem. They are found in mushrooms and tomatoes and parmesan cheese. But when they are freed from the protein they become a so-called Excito-toxin. According to research done by a prominent Neurosurgeon, Excito-toxins hyper-excite your brain cells to the point where they die," said Niblet. "And earlier studies showed them to cause retinal damage in rodents, and lesions on the Hypothalamus."

"Legions on the Hippopotamus?" exclaimed Olivia.

"No, lesions or sores on the Hypothalamus," answered Niblet.

"What is a Hypothalamus?" asked Wesa.

"It is a region of your brain that controls many bodily functions, including body temperature, thirst, hunger, and sleep," responded Niblet. "Many other studies have linked the overuse of Glutamates with the rise in obesity. Like, HFCS, it upsets the fine balance between the hormones that regulate hunger. But it is very widely used a flavor enhancer, because it can make even awful concoctions taste great."

"Artificially Delicious. Right," chirped Olivia.

"Yep, that's it," agreed Giuliana.

"Many people think that MSG sensitivity is simply an allergy, however, based on studies of the immune system response to MSG, we know the reactions are in response to a toxic substance. There are certain people who are acutely sensitive and can actually go into a coma after eating them, but more common reactions are much milder and sometimes go unnoticed," said Niblet.

"But they are now hiding the glutamates, aren't they Niblet? Dad said that since most people know to look out for MSG, the manufacturers have started using other "Free Glutamates" that people are not familiar with. Did you know that there are dozens of ways to hide Free Glutamates, such as Pea Protein Extract, Hydrolyzed Vegetable Protein, etc. so you have to do your homework and read your labels if you want to avoid it," declared Giuliana.

"Right," agreed Niblet. "I have found four or five of them in a single product. The important thing to know is that they are not labeled on the nutrient panel so you have to read the ingredients listing in order to find them."

"You said these were Excito-Toxins Niblet. Isn't aspartame an Excito-Toxin as well?" asked Giuliana.

"Wow Giuliana, where did you learn that?" asked Niblet.

"I remember Dad talking about it. That neurologist's book you mentioned detailed the dangers of these ingredients," answered Giuliana.

"Yes, Aspartame contains aspartic acid which acts on the same part of your brain as the Glutamates," remarked Niblet.

"Oh yeah, the Hippotomus, right?" joked Olivia.

"The Hypothalamus!!!" demanded Giuliana. "Wait, Niblet, you are saying that these chemicals are working together to damage the same part of your brain. There is definitely something wrong with this picture."

"There certainly is. And there have been many crusaders that have tried to warn the public and change the rules so that these chemicals would be more clearly labeled and disclosed, but the governing bodies have decided that there is not a problem so nothing has been done," agreed Niblet.

"The best was to change the way things are being made is to make better choices. If we choose foods that do not contain all of these harmful and dangerous additives then industry will provide us with better choices," said Giuliana.

"And if enough people decide that this it is important and ask for better choices then everyone will have a better chance to be healthy. But it starts with us. We have to educate ourselves and we have to eat foods not chemicals!" Wesa chimed in.

"That is right, kids," said Niblet. "Once we create our list, we can distribute the label decoder book to all of our friends. We can create a movement. Why don't we call it "Coalition for a Chemical Free Lunch?"

"That sounds grand. But who is this so-called coalition?" asked Giuliana.

"I think it's us for right now," said Wesa. "But that does not mean that it has to stay that way."

"That is right children," agreed Niblet. "Remember, you have the power to make a difference. You just need to believe in yourselves and you will find the way."

"Niblet, Right now I am going to find the way to bed, because I am tired," commented Wesa.

"Me too," said Olivia.

"Tomorrow is another day. We have done all of the hard work. Tomorrow we will continue with the Nutrient Facts Panel and unravel the mystery of Wesa's problem. I am sure that you can see now that there are a lot of potential problems hiding in the "foods' that we eat. We need to make sure that we avoid those problems so that we can be healthy," Niblet summed up.

So the girls began to get ready for bed and Wesa called his mom and asked her to come pick him up. His head was filled to the brim with all that Niblet had taught them. He didn't speak with his mom the whole ride home as he went over all the crazy details from the day. That night he had trouble sleeping because he couldn't wait to begin again in the morning.

8 BREAKING DOWN THE LABEL

The next day, Wesa rose early and got ready quickly. Even though it was a Sunday and he usually slept in, he was eager to get back to work. This business of decoding labels was very cool even though it was a bit confusing. He was hoping to get a better handle on the concepts today. He began to wonder how we had arrived at such a funny place in the world of food. The more junk food and non-foods that the manufacturers produce the worse off everyone seemed to get. He knew that each person had to take responsibility for what they consumed, but did not see how that could be done if very few people actually understood what was in the food.

Wesa was very grateful that Olivia and Giuliana were helping him, and Niblet had proved to be an angel in disguise. With all his knowledge, they were going to create a rulebook for the other children in the neighborhood. If all of the kids were reading labels and making better choices it would be a lot easier to go along. It would be hard to stay away from junk food if all of the other kids were eating it.

Wesa traipsed down the stairs and into the kitchen. He was hungry for breakfast, so he went into the pantry to have a look around. Brightly colored boxes claiming all types of health benefits stacked floor to ceiling. Low Fat, High Fiber, Cholesterol Free, Zero Trans fats, Fortified with Minerals and Vitamins the boxes shouted at him. But he knew better. Those claims were nothing more than a showman's diversion. They get you looking one way and fool you as you gawk. He decided that there wasn't any "real" food in the pantry so he slowly and sadly shut the door. He looked around for the fruit basket and grabbed a banana and an apple. "I don't have to read the ingredients on these," he thought as he walked toward the garage. He dug around in the basket for his bicycle helmet, and then grabbed his bike and rode off toward Olivia and Giuliana's house.

As he peddled he kept thinking about food and especially growing food. Professor B had started a nice community garden at the University. Perhaps they could get one going at the school, Wesa thought. That way, we would be 100% sure about how our food is grown and processed. He was going to have to speak with Professor B about this. If he was able to get a garden planted at the University, we should be able to get one planted at school.

As he pulled up to Giuliana and Olivia's house he realized that it was actually quite early. In all his excitement he had not even bothered to look at the clock. He knew that Giuliana wouldn't be up yet but he went ahead and knocked on the door anyhow. He was excited and determined. This was his best chance to get back to his old self again. And he knew that he would be able to help others just like him, including his parents.

Waiting at the door, he heard a bark and then a bang, "That sounds like Olivia and MooMoo," he thought. As the door opened his suspicions were confirmed. There was Olivia in her PJ's with the goofy dog in tow. Wesa was usually scared of dogs, but MooMoo was an exception. She began to lick Wesa's hand as he reached to pet her and Olivia laughed.

"Come on in," Olivia said. "Giuliana's not up yet, but we can play with Niblet."

"Cool, maybe we can get started. I am very anxious," said Wesa. "I really want to figure out what I have been eating and learn to make better choices."

"Don't worry Wesa; you are going to do it. Niblet will repeat it as many times as it takes," declared Olivia. "And once you get it, you can shout it from the hills if you want."

"What do you mean 'shout it from the hills'?" Wesa inquired.

"I mean, SPREAD THE WORD. Sheesh, haven't you ever heard that one before?" asked Olivia.

"Nope, but it makes sense now! We are going to 'shout from the hills' and give copies of our decoder to all of the kids at school. Before long, we will make a big difference!" exclaimed Wesa.

In the back of his mind he was still thinking about the school garden. "Gardens will be the next step," he thought to himself. "And I am going to take it!" he resolved solemnly.

They walked down the hall and looked in on Giuliana.

"Dead to the world," Olivia said. "She will be up later. Don't bother trying to wake her, it never works. She was probably up until about two in the morning reading. She always does that."

"Let's go talk to Niblet," Wesa whispered.

"Yeppers, I will go get him. Meet me in the office," Olivia responded loudly; in stark contrast to Wesa's gentle tone.

Wesa entered the office and sat down at the desk in front of the computer. He opened his email and looked at the notes that Giuliana had sent him from their discussions yesterday. "Wow," he thought. "This is a lot of information." He knew he was going to have to find a simple way to present this. Otherwise, it is too much for most kids, especially the ones eating all the toxic garbage. With their brains scrambled like this morning's breakfast, Wesa and the girls were going to have to be really clever to get the information across.

As Wesa sat there and thought, he began to doodle. He drew a picture of a head full of scrambled eggs. "Funny," he thought. "Perhaps we can use pictures for the code-book showing the effects of each ingredient. That way you could just glance at the picture and know what the problem was. We could have a picture of a big fat head for things that make you fat and one with a big lump on it for things that were carcinogenic. This was getting good," he thought. "Then we could put the evidence and studies up on the Coalition website, so people can learn more about it if they are interested."

When Olivia strolled in with Niblet on her shoulder, Wesa could barely control his excitement.

"Niblet," Wesa cried, "I think I've got it."

Niblet jumped up on the keyboard and slippedy-slide and a clackety-clack he swiftly responded to Wesa. "What did you "get" Wesa?" Niblet asked.

"I "Got" the best idea for the de-coder. I got it!" Wesa bubbled with enthusiasm. "We will use pictures which symbolize the effects of each ingredient, so the children can easily see if something is harmful or not. They can go to the website and learn about the potential effects of these ingredients if they want to learn more or educate their parents."

"That is a great idea Wesa. Kind of like the old Skull and Crossbones on the poisons right?" asked Niblet, sliding around the computer.

"That's exactly what I said earlier," said Olivia

"Pictures certainly make lasting impressions," said Niblet. "In Brazil and other countries they put real pictures of the body parts ravaged by the effects smoking on cigarettes packages. The intent is to deter smoking. If each child were to write down all of the unhappy faces associated with their favorite junk foods they probably would think twice about eating them."

"That's a totally rad idea. I will draw the pictures," said Olivia.

"The kids will be able to de-code each food item using the different faces. As they read the ingredients they will translate the recipe by drawing the face which corresponds with each ingredient. When there is a good ingredient they'll add a happy face. That way, just one look at the de-coded version will tell them if they should be eating something or not!" said Wesa.

Just then, Giuliana walked in, bleary eyed and tired but with a gleam of excitement on her face. She could tell they were all up to something and she wanted in.

"What's going down guys? What are you doing over here so early Wesa?" asked Giuliana. "And come to think of it, what am I doing up?"

` "I just wanted to get started, so I rushed over here early. Then I had the greatest idea," said Wesa.

Wesa excitedly explained the coding system that he had conceived, going over all the details. When he finished, he spoke softly, "What do you think," he said.

"That is a totally rockin' idea," Giuliana exclaimed. "Let's start by de-coding the labels from your pantry. One good look at those results should be enough to stop you from eating that stuff.

Let's start with that label we used an example yesterday."

So, while Olivia grabbed some paper and began to draw her own pictures, Wesa and Giuliana focused on the ingredient statement from yesterday's lecture with Niblet. They decided to simply use happy and sad faces for the first translation of the label.

.

ENRICHED FLOUR (Simple Carbohydrate), CORN SYRUP (Added Sugar),

HIGH FRUCTOSE CORN SYRUP (Added Sugar), DEXTROSE (Added Sugar),

SOYBEAN AND PALM OIL (WITH TBHQ FOR FRESHNESS) (Preservative),

SUGAR (Added Sugar), CRACKER MEAL, WHEAT STARCH, SALT, DRIED BLUEBERRIES, DRIED GRAPES, DRIED APPLES, CORNSTARCH, LEAVENING(BAKING SODA, SODIUM ACID PYROPHOSPHATE, MONOCALCIUM PHOSPHATE), CITRIC ACID, CORN CEREAL, GELATIN, PARTIALLY HYDROGENATED SOYBEAN OIL†, MODIFIED CORN STARCH, NATURAL AND ARTIFICIAL BLUEBERRY FLAVOR, MODIFIED WHEAT STARCH, SOY LECITHIN, TRICALCIUM PHOSPHATE, XANTHAN GUM, CARAMEL COLOR, COLOR ADDED, NATURAL AND ARTIFICIAL FLAVOR, TURMERIC EXTRACT, RED #40, VITAMIN A PALMITATE, NIACINAMIDE, REDUCED IRON, BLUE #2, BLUE #1, PYRIDOXINE HYDROCHLORIDE (VITAMIN B6), RIBOFLAVIN (VITAMIN B2), THIAMIN HYDROCHLORIDE (VITAMIN B1), FOLIC ACID. †LESS THAN 0.5g TRANS FAT PER SERVING

They didn't get far before they realized there were already too many sad faces. They had reached the sixth ingredient and hadn't even drawn one smile yet.

"Look for yourself! This is not food. I see four different types of sugar and simple carbohydrates along with some preserved oil as the first six ingredients. We didn't even get to plethora of artificial colors and flavors listed at the end, and we already have way too many frowns. Your idea for breaking down the ingredients is great, but we also need to talk about how to examine the rest of the label. You will find that the Nutrition Facts panel and the rest of the writing on the package are helpful, but should ALWAYS lead you back to the actual ingredients. Since not all calories are the same, nor are all fats, carbohydrates, or sugars. You must read the ingredients to determine where they came from," Niblet insisted firmly.

"Yesterday we put together a sufficient list of problem ingredients, so you will know what to look for when you read that part of the label," said Niblet. "Now, let's focus on where most people put their attention: The Nutrition Facts Panel."

"Niblet, let me try to explain it. You can help me if I get confused, Ok?" Giuliana butted in.

"Hey, Olivia, grab those crackers that were on the table in the living room would you?" asked Giuliana.

"Why do I have to do everything?" snapped Olivia.

"No worries, I'll get it Giuliana," Wesa said gently.

Wesa walked down the hall to the living room and grabbed the box of crackers. He flipped it over and gazed at the nutrient panel. It sure looked like a lot of information. "Am I going to understand this? Do I really need to know this just to be healthy?" thought Wesa. As he walked back into the office he was not overly excited any longer. This was not going to be so easy.

It was laid out like this:

Nutrition Facts

Serving Size 1 grams (56g)
Serving Per Container 1

Amount Per Serving	
Calories 150	
	% Daily Values*
Total Fat 7g	**11%**
Saturated Fat 1g	**5%**
Trans Fat 0g	
Cholesterol 130mg	**43%**
Sodium 90mg	**4%**
Total Carbohydrate 20g	**7%**
Dietary Fiber 1g	**4%**
Sugars 13g	
Protein 2g	**4%**

*Percent Daily Values are based on a 2,000 calorie diet.

Giuliana noticed Wesa's glum look and tried to cheer him up. "Hey, Wesa what did the big tomato say to the small tomato right before they were run over by a car?"

"I don't know," said Wesa

"Ketchup," giggled Oliva.

"That was my joke, Olivia." Said Giuliana.

"Funny," said Wesa, "but I am confused. Am I ever going to get it?"

"Don't worry, we will keep working on this until we have got it down cold. That's the only way we can help you, not to mention all of the other children. We must become experts. The children of the neighborhood are counting on us, even if they don't know it yet." Said Giuliana.

Niblet jumped in. "Yes Wesa. We will take all the time that is necessary. This is critical for your health, and your future," Niblet agreed.

"Alright," Wesa said, his voicing gaining a bit of confidence. "Let's do this thing. Where do we begin?"

"Listed at the top of the panel, you will see Serving Size and number of servings in the container. It doesn't help to know the nutrient value of a serving if you don't know how many servings there are in the container. A serving can be a whole package or just a small portion of it. The values they are giving are specific for the serving size, so if you eat 5 servings of the food and the nutrient panel says 100 calories per serving than you ate 500 calories. Do you understand?" Giuliana began, smartly and proudly.

"I think so. The first two numbers at the top are the size of the product and how many of them there are in the package. But the nutrient values can look artificially low because they are broken down into minute serving sizes. You need to know how many of the servings you are eating to know how many calories, fats, proteins, etc. that you are getting. So where does it go from there," Wesa responded.

Calories:

"First on the Nutrition Facts panel is Calories," said Olivia smartly.

"And what are calories?" asked Niblet.

"They are a general scientific measure of energy," Giuliana chimed in. "In this case it is a measure of the energy stored in food. Specifically, a gram of Fat has 9 calories while a gram of Protein or

Carbohydrates have 4 calories each. That means fats have more than twice the number of calories, or energy stored, per gram as Protein or Carbohydrates."

"Excellent Giuliana. You got that one down. Furthermore, calories are the primary manner most people use to account for how much food they are eating. The USDA recommends a total of 2200 calories per day for an active child of your age. Have you heard of "counting calories" Wesa?" asked Niblet.

"Sure, hasn't everyone? My mother always looks at the panel and buys things that are low calorie. But you said yesterday that empty calories can make the body crave more and more food in order to get the nutrients it needs. And this leads to increased consumption and weight gain," said Wesa. "Isn't that what you said Niblet?"

"Again, Wesa, you are right. Empty Calories are those that are highly processed and stripped of their nutrients," said Niblet. "So the idea of simply counting calories is not enough. In Colin Campbell's famous work "The China Study," the Chinese people consumed almost twice the number of calories recommended by the USDA, but they didn't have an obesity problem or the myriad related diseases. Their diet consisted primarily of unprocessed plant foods, which are Nutrient Dense. So the idea is that our focus should be on eating whole foods, not just calorie counting. Sadly, the contemporary urban Chinese have largely adopted our processed diet in the past decade and now suffer similar rates of obesity and disease."

"So, do I need to watch my calories, or not?" asked Wesa.

"Well, yes and no. If you eat whole foods, whole grains, and mostly plants your body will naturally regulate itself; so, watching calories is not the most critical thing. One thousand calories of brown rice is nothing like one thousand calories of gummy bears to your body, so simply watching the number of calories misses the point. Eating the brown rice will satiate your hunger and deliver nutrients, while eating the gummy worms will give you a sugar rush, followed by a crash, and leave you craving real food," said Niblet.

"So, even if you look at the number of calories, you must always ask yourself, "Calories from what?" said Giuliana. "Which means….what, Wesa."

"Oh, I know, I know," said Olivia.

"Ok, Olivia, you can answer this one," said Niblet.

"It means that even if you know how many calories there are, you still need to read the ingredient statement to find out where the calories come from," said Olivia.

"I believe that is right," Said Wesa. "Isn't it, Niblet?"

"That is correct. You must always read the ingredient panel to find out what you are eating. The caloric counts, grams of carbohydrates and fats, etc. can only be understood after reading the ingredients," said Niblet. "There are no short cuts to good health. If you don't want to read the label, than you shouldn't eat the food."

"You probably mean, "That which is PURPORTED to be food,"" Giuliana interjected loudly.

"Getting a little excited by this Giuliana?" asked Wesa.

"She is, and you should be too. Look at what happened to your health in just six short months. If you don't learn these lessons, your future will be full of ailments, trips to the doctor, medications and whatnot. If you do learn this stuff, you can count on regaining that razor sharp intellect and those fleet feet you always had. The choice is yours," said Niblet.

"I am in. 100%. OK?" said Wesa.

"OK," said Niblet. "Let's get back to work. What is next Olivia?"

Fats:

"Fats!" she yelled.

"Ok, what do we know about fats kids?" asked Niblet.

"They are not good for you. That is for sure." Said Olivia

Olivia was about to continue when Niblet jumped in. "Whoa, hold your horses little-missie. Did you say fats were not good for you?"

"Yep, everyone knows that. My best friend told me. They

only eat low-fat things because her dad has high cholesterol," said Olivia.

"That is what my parents do too," Wesa agreed.

"Well, that is a very common misconception. In fact your body desperately needs fats and your brain is those most needy of all. The USDA recommendation for Fats is around 73 grams per day, which is easily reached with today's foods," said Niblet. "However, the China Study along with substantial new evidence shows definitively that animal proteins are much more the culprit in high cholesterol and heart disease than the fats. Certain fats, such as omega 3's are especially good for the brain and most Americans are deficient in them."

"The Nutrition Facts Panel breaks FAT down into Total Fat, Saturated Fat and Trans-fats, which each come from a different source," said Niblet.

"What is the difference between them?" asked Giuliana.

"Saturated Fat is primarily from animal sources, whereas trans-fats are delivered through the Hydrogenation process, which we discussed yesterday," Niblet replied.

"Right. Making bad fats from good ones. I remember," said Wesa.

"The other fats come from plant sources. As with everything else, you must read the ingredients to find out where they come from and see if they are hiding anything like trans-fats or one of the Letter Preservatives in the oil," Niblet said firmly.

"I got it. I got it! We MUST "read the ingredients" to know what we are eating," said Wesa.

"The panel also shows the percentage of the total calories from fat, and many people avoid things that are high in this regard. But by doing this, they miss the essential fats found in nuts and seeds, which are very high in fat as a percentage of the total calories. Again, you need to read the ingredient panel and find out where the fats are coming from. Cashews and chicken nuggets have similar percentages of calories from fat but everyone knows they are not the same," Niblet implored.

"And I guess we are especially looking for Hydrogenated Oil or Partially Hydrogenated Oils, because those are on our list of problem ingredients, right Niblet?" asked Wesa.

"Yes, although in 2006 they created a place to disclose grams of Trans-Fats on the label, they can still be lurking if they occur in small amounts so you must look for the word Hydrogenated. Remember, this is the worst type of fat you can ingest so you want to be sure that you avoid it at all costs," said Niblet.

"The best types of fats for our health come from plants, right Niblet." Giuliana asked smartly.

"Not quite, Giuliana. In my studies I have found a lot of recent evidence suggesting there are beneficial compounds in animal fats that were previously unknown. But that is a good "general idea". And It goes along with what we already know from Michael Pollan: "Eat Food, Mostly Plants, Not Too Much." To recap, what do we need to do?"

"READ the Ingredient LABEL!" All three shouted in Unison.

Niblet jumped back and covered his ears. He flashed a sheepish grin at Wesa and thought to himself. "I think they are getting it."

"Now you seem to understand. We can't be sure that we are eating foods, "mostly plants" unless we read the ingredients. Even if the Nutrient Panel looks great to a "Nutritionist" the actual "food" that delivers those nutrients might contain many things that are terrible and that should not be consumed under any circumstances," said Niblet.

Carbohydrates:

"I guess the next thing, Carbohydrates, will be the same as well?" asked Wesa.

"You know it Wesa," said Giuliana. "Carbohydrates come primarily from sugars, fiber, and starch. But they are not all the same. Stripped flours and whole grain flours both contain carbohydrates but your body processes them very differently. Stripped carbohydrates like white bread are treated exactly like sugar in the body creating short term energy spikes followed by a crash. So regardless of how many carbohydrates are listed we must know the source. Do they come from simple sugars or complex carbohydrates? Remember Gummy worms or Brown rice?"

"So we must read the ingredient label to be certain that we are getting our carbohydrates from whole food sources?" queried Wesa

"Right again, Wesa. The USDA recommends between 250 and 325 grams of carbohydrates per day, or up to 65% of your total calories. But lately Carbohydrates have gotten a very bad name, and many people avoid them. But they are very important, and we need them more than we need anything else. The real problem is the EMPTY CARBOHYDRATES we discussed earlier; foods with little nutritional value," said Niblet. "Let's move on."

"We are down to the last four things on the nutrient panel," said Olivia. "Cholesterol, Sodium, Sugar and Protein. Niblet, what in the world is Cholesterol? It sounds funny."

Cholesterol:

"Cholesterol is produced by the liver and is another thing that we need. When there is too much in the body it circulates in the blood and can cause heart and other problems. It is primarily from animal sources, but as we discussed earlier, many people blame animal proteins and refined sugar and not dietary cholesterol as the cause of the ailments," said Niblet.

"So if you limit animal and refined carbohydrate intake, especially sugar, you will be naturally reducing your risk of high cholesterol?" questioned Giuliana.

"You could say that Giuliana. The USDA recommends that you keep your daily cholesterol intake below 300mg per day, which is about the amount in a single egg. Not very much. In order to meet this goal, you will need to limit your intake of animal products in general" Niblet responded.

"Evidence points to sugar as a primary cause of high cholesterol. In fact, Dad told me the Sugar Association won some huge award from the Public Relations Industry in the 70's for their campaign to deflect and counter growing evidence that their product was a primary culprit in the rise of heart disease?" Giuliana shot back.

"That is right. Evidence has and does point to sugar and other simple carbohydrates as the primary culprit in elevated blood cholesterol and heart disease and we have already discussed that. But limiting your dietary cholesterol to the ranges suggested by the USDA will not be hard if you are limiting your overall animal intake, so let's move on. Remember, cholesterol intake is important, but if you are eating the way we are describing you will be fine. What did you say was next, Olivia, Sodium right?" asked Niblet.

Sodium:

"You got it. What's with the Sodium anyway? Is it good for you?" Olivia inquired.

"Sodium is very important for your health, but not in the high levels found in foods today. You get most of your sodium from Salt and other flavor enhancers, which are in everything these days. If you eat processed foods often, than you are undoubtedly be consuming far too much Sodium," said Niblet. "It is important to keep your sodium intake below 2400mg per day, and this is very hard to achieve if you are eating a lot of processed foods. But, if you stick with whole foods that are minimally processed, sodium will never be a problem for you. Again, you must keep an eye on this one Wesa." Niblet implored.

"What is next Olivia?" asked Niblet. "Are you looking at the nutrient panel?"

Sugar:

"Yep, I am looking at it. Next up is Sugar Niblet. And I know that sugar gives you cavities." Said Olivia.

"Well, yes, Sugar can give you cavities. But the greatest problem with sugar today is similar to sodium. We eat too much of it. We do need sugar, but not nearly as much as we are typically eating. The World Health recommendation for sugar is less than 50 grams per day or about 10% of your total calories, and recent US recommendations are even lower. But High Fructose Corn Syrup and other sugars are good for preservation, so manufacturers use them everywhere. Remember, there were four types of sugar in the first six ingredients of the item we reviewed earlier. As a result people eat way too much of them," said Niblet.

"Hold On! I was looking at one of those 20oz bottles of Coke the other day and it had 65 grams of sugar," said Giuliana.

"That is more than our entire daily allowance in one beverage. That could not be right, could it?"

"Actually, it is Giuliana. Worst of all, sugar has been proven to have a prominent role in the cause of Obesity and its related diseases such as Hypertension, Metabolic Syndrome, Heart disease, etc. And as you can tell by your soda example, Americans consume WAY too much Sugar. Period. Everyday products like yogurt, oatmeal, or "protein bars" that appear healthy are often heavily laden with sugar. You must look at the nutrient panel and keep your sugar consumption within the guidelines. But you must also read the ingredients, because, and this is VERY IMPORTANT WESA…artificial sweeteners are commonly used in conjunction with sugar to reduce the number of sugar grams listed on the Nutrition Facts Panel. They don't measure artificial sweeteners, just sugar. BUT it doesn't make sense to reduce our sugar intake if we are going to replace it with something far worse like aspartame or acelfame-k."

"So, we need to look at the nutrient panel but we also must look at the ingredient statement to see how the food is made," Wesa replied.

"Of course. Raisins or other dried fruits are high in sugar, but that is different from refined and processed sugars that are added. We need to keep an eye out for added sugars as well as artificial flavors and sweeteners that don't appear on the Nutrient Facts panel at all. This is getting sort of redundant because it is the same with everything, right Wesa?" asked Niblet rhetorically.

"You got it my little professor, you must read the ingredients." Wesa shot back.

"We are down to Protein and then we are done with this?" Olivia said excitedly.

"Not quite," Said Niblet. "After we talk about protein, we are going to discuss various techniques food companies use so that we can better understand the label. Remember, each revelation by the public regarding a problem ingredient or tactic causes industry to make changes. Sometimes the changes genuinely improve the food, but "change" can also be a way to hide the truth."

"Like the way MSG is hiding in so many foods right now?" Asked Wesa.

"Yes, that is a good example. Many people are aware that MSG can create adverse reactions so they specifically look for it in the ingredient listing. But since they don't know that "hydrolyzed protein" is essentially the same thing, industry will use that instead. They call it "Cleaning Up" their labels," said Niblet.

"You said "Cleaning Up" their labels but not cleaning up the foods?" Giuliana interjected.

"Uh huh, I did. Until everyone begins to read labels, educate themselves, and demand products that are actually cleaner and healthier, the shell game will continue," Niblet said pessimistically.

Protein:

"So, what about protein, Niblet? Protein is for your muscles, isn't it Giu Giu?" Olivia began.

"I think so. Is that right Niblet?" replied Giuliana.

"Proteins are critical for growth, and some of them are not produced by your body, so they must be gotten from your foods. The USDA recommends between 10 and 35 percent of your total calories from protein, but many nutritionists believe that 35% is way too high. You can get protein from both animal and vegetable sources, but in the USA we rely mostly on cheap meat," said Niblet.

"Is that bad?" Wesa asked. "We have been eating quite a bit of lean meat and poultry at the direction of our Doctor."

"According to Dr. Campbell's research, and Dean Ornish's, the diseases killing Americans are caused by eating too much Animal Proteins. Dr. Campbell suggests keeping your intake of animal proteins to no more than 8% of your total calories. In his extensive studies, he demonstrated that over consumption of animal proteins, not fats, to be the most problematic. So we must watch our animal protein intake and try to get much of our protein from plants." Said Niblet.

"I remember what Dad always said. It is either a Plant or an Animal. That is the distinction, not whether it is fish, chicken, or anything else. Animals are animals, plants are plants," Giuliana chimed in. "Right Niblet?"

"Very good, but remember, we should not replace animal protein with Hexane laden GMO Soy proteins either. Many people eat them to avoid meat and think they are healthy because they are plant based. Everything from Veggie Burgers to Protein Bars are using this cheap and dangerous protein because people think that they will build more muscle or be healthier if they increase their protein. What we should look for instead are whole grains, legumes and nuts rather than highly processed and residue laden soy," said Niblet.

"You mean you don't need to eat meat to be healthy?" asked Wesa.

"That is exactly right. Dad has told me that some of the greatest athletes in the world are actually Vegan, even some Big Ginormous Football Players," said Giuliana.

"Ginormous Vegans, sounds terrifying," said Olivia.

"Vegan just means that don't eat anything that comes from an animal, even milk, cheese and eggs." said Giuliana, herself a vegetarian, but far from Vegan.

"Wesa, I think what Giuliana is saying is that we don't need as much protein as most people think and we can actually get most of the protein we need from plants. But we aren't saying you can't have animals in your diet, just that you should limit them. As I said, grains, beans and nuts are excellent sources of protein that are extremely healthy. And 8% of your total 2000 calories or 160 calories worth of protein is 40 grams which is between 5 and six ounces of meat or other animal product per day. Now, if you are also eating yogurt, milk, cheese, and other dairy products, than this number will add up quickly. You will have to read the ingredient statement to find out where the protein is derived. Again, animals are animals, plants are plants. That is the distinction here." said Niblet.

"We keep saying the same thing over and over. You have to read the Nutrient Panel but you cannot simply stop there. You must also read the ingredient statement to see what is actually being done with the food / non-food." replied Wesa.

"Exactly Wesa, both the Nutrient Panel and the ingredients must be read to understand what you are eating, which brings us to a couple of things that we should know about food labeling," said Niblet.

Tricks of the Trade:

"One of the astonishing things about the Nutrition Facts Panel is what is not listed," said Niblet.

"What exactly do you mean Niblet?" asked Olivia.

"Well, the nutrients listed on the Nutrition Facts Panel were only discovered in the last century. Now research is uncovering many other nutrients in the food that we are not counting. These phyto-nutrients are processed out of the whole foods but they aren't measured or listed so nobody knows they are missing them. Moreover, there is no requirement to label the levels of artificial preservatives, flavors, enhancers, or residues. Remember that man we discussed earlier who worked so hard to have the levels of Free Glutamates listed on the panel? He has been fighting for more than 20 years to make that happen because Glutamates represent such an acute risk to his health, but to no avail," Niblet responded.

"That is why the Nutrition Facts Panel for things that are stripped and bleached and flavored look very similar to those made with whole foods." said Giuliana smartly.

"Exactly. We know many additional nutrients as well as residues are present, but they do not appear on the panel; perhaps intentionally, perhaps not. So, once again I say, you must read the ingredient declaration and eat Whole Foods. That is the only way you know you are getting all of the nutrients that nature intended," Niblet continued.

"What else can you tell us about the ingredient listing?" asked Wesa.

The Ingredient Listing:

"Here are some basics," said Niblet.

"Ingredients must be listed in order of predominance. So the first few ingredients will give you a good understanding of what the basic building blocks of the "Food" product are. But, there are ways of tricking the consumer," said Niblet.

"Yeah, I heard Dad talk about "ingredient stacking?" said Giuliana.

"Oh, that's where you get all your ingredients stacked and ready before you make the thing?" asked Olivia.

"Not hardly. Ingredient stacking is where you use several types of a similar ingredient so that none of them occurs as the most predominant. Remember there were 4 types of sugar in the first six ingredients of that product earlier. If they had used just one type of sugar, it would appear before the Flour and everyone would know quickly that the food was primarily sugar. So they break the sweeteners down into four different types and thusly layer them in. That is why you must read all of the ingredients, and avoid added sugars, preservatives, etc."

"Do you have to read the entire label, Niblet?" asked Olivia.

"Of course you must. There is a point in the ingredient declaration where it now says, "Less than 2% of the following:", but just because the concentration is less than 2% does not mean it is OK. You frequently find very potent ingredients in this section; ingredients which can affect you even at very small doses. There is recent evidence that the old idea that the "danger is in the dose" is wrong and that micro amounts of certain widely used chemicals are wreaking havoc on our bodies. The manufacturer is saying, "It's just a tiny amount, so you can stop reading here." But, the devil is always in the details." Niblet lectured.

"So, do you think some manufactures are deliberately trying to confuse the consumer?" asked Giuliana.

"That seems to be the case Giuliana. But once you read

labels for a time, you will see that manufacturers use the same problem ingredients over and over. You will soon begin to identify the companies that do and don't use the ingredients you are trying so hard to avoid. You will develop loyalty for brand or product you trust, but you must be ever-vigilant as things can change over time."

"Aren't we done yet?" said Olivia. "I am hungry and all this talk about food is killing me."

"Well, I guess I can finish with the following: Health claims are made to sell food, not necessarily to provide healthy choices. Fortified garbage is still garbage, albeit scented and flavored. In the same way, there is plenty of ORGANIC junk food loaded with sodium, fats and sugars. In fact the other day I saw a box of Organic Vegan Jelly Beans. Are those healthy?" Niblet queried.

"Of course not!" The children replied in unison.

"Remember, there are no health claims on apples but we know what the ancient wisdom says about them. If a food product needs to claim to be healthy, something is probably not right about it. Sort of like the old saying, "If you have to tell people how good you are, you are probably not that good." Whole foods are almost always obviously so, and if you have any doubt, what do you do?"

"READ THE LABEL. If you don't read it, you shouldn't eat it!" they shouted once again!

9 SHOUTING FROM THE HILLS

Wesa had been a bit dumbfounded by Niblet's lecture, but the more he thought about it, the more it made sense. In Africa he did not have as much variety of foods, but everything was local and made fresh. It did not need chemicals because it did not have to last long. It was very likely that Niblet was right about the additives and his health. The things that he had been eating were very different from what he was accustomed to and what would be natural for a human being. He was beginning to have hope that changing his diet would return his life to normal. After all, those were some incredibly scary things that Niblet told him about food additives. And something Niblet didn't mention was that in product testing, where it was even done, additives were tested one at a time. Today people are now consuming many of these devilish additives at once, something like a perfect storm for bad health. "Who in the world can honestly say that the foods with these additives are completely safe?" Wesa pondered.

Wesa needed a plan to change his diet, but he knew he

could not do it without his parents. They were like so many others who desperately wanted to eat right and be healthy, but were completely confused by the system and over-stimulated by the additives. He knew that his parents would go along if he could just get them to look at the evidence. He decided that his family would be the first to get the decoder, and they would use it together in the supermarket to make better food choices. He knew they would go along because of all the hard work the kids had done on it. So, Wesa collected his wits, along with all of Giuliana's emails and crafted the first draft of the decoder. He decided to simplify it greatly. He would simply use a Happy Face for good ingredients, and a Sad Face for bad ones. It really made no difference if the additive was carcinogenic or otherwise harmful; either way they were bad. And not everyone would be able to draw all of the different faces when they decoded their labels. So sticking with the Happy and Sad faces would be perfect.

Wesa decided to give his parents the decoder right after dinner. If he could convince them of the veracity of the evidence he was going to get them to make a pledge to eat only real "foods." He was ready to promise anything, if only they would go along. And he knew one thing for certain; it is very hard to ignore the truth if you have educated yourself. Once the proverbial genie was out of the bottle, it would be very hard to put back.

And so it went. That night after dinner as they were clearing the dishes, Wesa said to his mother, "Hey mom, do you know what I have been doing with Giuliana and Olivia this past weekend?"

"I thought you were playing with that funny little rodent of theirs," his Mother replied.

"Well, we did play some, but mostly we were learning about food and how food is made," Wesa continued.

"And who exactly was teaching you about food," asked his Father. "Are they qualified to be telling you what to eat? Are they a doctor? After all, you have some serious health issues?"

"Niblet was teaching us. He is a real Scientist. He helped me and the girls discover the many chemical additives I have been eating and how they could be harming me. We went through the pantry and freezer, copied all of the labels and "De-Coded" them. I was shocked by all of the strange ingredients that we found. But I was more surprised by how they can damage your health."

"The Mouse is a scientist?" his father inquired quizzically. "Now you are stretching the truth just a bit too much. I will not tolerate dishonesty Wesa!"

"I am not lying father. It is true! Professor B really did teach Niblet all of his secrets, but Niblet hid his abilities because he was afraid. Then when he found out about my health issues he decided to help me. He brushed up on every single ingredient and showed me and the girls exactly what the detrimental health effects of each one were. I thought you wouldn't believe me, so we did the project in secret. But now the hard work is done. We created a de-coder to help people understand what they are eating. See for yourself," pleaded Wesa. "Please, just look at it."

Wesa handed to de-coder over to his father who began to peruse the information. In very short time he looked up from the page and just stared at Wesa in disbelief.

"If this information is correct, it is no wonder that you are not well. In fact, this may explain some of the issues that your mother and I have had over the years. I can honestly tell you Wesa, that I had no idea," said Wesa's Father.

"It is correct!" Wesa stammered. "Niblet showed us all of the evidence, and he put them up on a blog called www.chemicalfreelunch.com"

"Well, I guess that settles it. Once we confirm this information is correct, we are going to eliminate these ingredients from our diet. It may sound radical, but once you have definitive information like this in your hands, only a fool would ignore it," said Wesa's Mother.

And since they were not fools, but well-meaning parents, they did not ignore it. They took the list to the market every time they went and began to learn which brands they could trust and which ones consistently used problem ingredients. As time went by, Wesa continued to eat healthful, whole foods, and his body did change. He got leaner and faster and began to excel again in his studies. And best of all, his parents had followed Niblet's advice as well. After a short time, they too were convinced that diet was fundamental for optimum health. They put down the Diet Sodas and "Lite" products and began to feel much better on a daily basis. They were so impressed and moved by the changes, that they began to think about how they could spread the word and help others to help themselves. "This was life-changing, and perhaps "World" changing," Wesa thought.

In the meantime, the kids had been hatching a plan. Since the most important thing, above all, was fresh, wholesome locally grown foods, then wouldn't a community school garden be the best first step? And who would be more qualified to start the garden than Professor B? And how far would it go toward repairing his reputation and standing in the community?

The first step was obvious. Professor B had to know about Niblet, although they suspected Dad had already spilled the beans. The professor was going to come asking about the software that Niblet bought on his account soon enough anyway. So the three children decided that they needed to go see Professor B. They would bring Niblet and ask the Professor to help them get the gardens planted and the code book distributed to the kids. They knew he could be a big help.

Wesa was certain that once Professor B knew the truth about Niblet, they would spill the beans about the Companies' dirty little secrets. Then nobody could deny the validity of their work. The obfuscation would end. After all, their game was up once the children had learned these lessons. With the code book and the gardens, futures would be changed forever. Illnesses and maladies affecting so many of them would be lifted by the simple magic of nature. Whooaa whaaoo, getting a little carried away you might think?

"Anything less than changing the world is Mickey Mouse to me," Dad used to say. But the kids never really got it until now. They could do something good, and right, and fight the good fight in front of them, or they could play around on their cell phones and watch TV as hope faded for so many children and friends. "The time for idol play had passed." Wesa determined.

So, it was decided. They would launch a dual initiative: code-books and gardens and good old fashioned "shouting from the hills". Eat this (garden), and don't eat this (code book) was the message. Excellent health could not be delivered in a pill, but gradually by eating whole foods and exercising. Of course, if you didn't eat the whole foods you really wouldn't feel like doing much of anything, so one thing was deeply reliant upon the other.

The following weekend was Professor B's birthday. The kids thought that it would be a great time to speak with him about Niblet. After all, it would make him so happy to know that he was right about that smart little rodent. And he would surely be serving up fresh vegetables from his garden. They would bring the code book and show them all the work that Niblet had done with them and then ask him to help them launch the community school gardens. It would be a great surprise. The kids were as excited as they were determined.

"We have to tell Professor B how much Niblet actually learned from him about science and chemicals and nutrition," said Wesa. "I think he saved my life."

"How many other children do you think we could we save

by getting the code books out there?" Olivia pondered aloud.

"It could be world changing," said Giuliana.

"I have an idea," said Olivia.

"I would say, "Don't Tell Me", but I know you will anyway." Giuliana shot back.

"Well, we should get Niblet to ask Professor B to help start the Gardens," Olivia went on. "He'll never refuse Niblet's request, that's for sure."

"That is a great idea," said Wesa. "Niblet will do that for us."

"Yeah, he will. We just have to bring the computer, you know, the one that is all loaded up with the software. That way Niblet can speak directly to him, just the way that Professor B had always imagined," said Giuliana. "Ok, so this Saturday, before the party, we will bring Niblet and the computer and "lay it all out on the table."" Giuliana said coyly, making quotation marks with her fingers to bring attention to the dual meaning.

With Saturday upon them, the girls woke early, which was never particularly easy for them unless they were excited. But this was like the first day of school and they had already called Wesa by 8:00am in the morning. He too was awake and ready. Giuliana called Wesa and challenged him, "I'll race you over to Professor B's house. Last one there has clean Niblet's cage for the next month!"

No sooner had Giuliana thrown down the gauntlet then

Wesa was out the kitchen door, into the garage, on his bicycle and down the road. They were about the same distance from Professor B's house so Wesa knew that any head-start he could manage would help. So off he went, racing down the road never thinking about the fact that if he did arrive first he was going to have some explaining to do!

Meanwhile, Giuliana and Olivia gathered up the computer and put it in their backpack. Then they grabbed Niblet and placed him in the little toy thingamagig that they carried him around in and put him in the handlebar basket. They weren't really going to race Wesa, because with his renewed health they really had no chance. And besides, they were carrying the computer and the wonder mouse, so it was better to take it easy. The girls really just wanted Wesa to be excited about his strength and speed so he would tell Dad and Professor B about what they had done.

As the girls had predicted, Wesa arrived like the wind in a flurry. He was excited and impatient for the day to proceed, but sitting out in front of Professor B's house all alone took some of the joy out of winning. He was too bashful to knock on the door all by himself, so he took a seat on the curb in front of the house and waited for the girls to arrive. From a window in the house, Professor B could see Wesa and he was puzzled. "How come Wesa is here so early, after all, the party doesn't start for hours, and if he's here, where are the girls?" he thought.

Certain that something was afoot, Professor B, sat patiently and waited for the events to unfold. He could see Wesa looking nervously down the street, obviously waiting for someone or something. "The girls probably put him up to this," Professor B thought. "I'll bet they are just about to make their appearance." And, as if on cue, the girls came rolling down the street, with intent but in no obvious hurry.

Wesa was excited. That was very clear. He jumped up from the curb and met the girls before they even stopped. "Where have you been?" he asked anxiously.

"Oh chillax, Wesa. We had to get Niblet's stuff and the computer. Besides, we knew we couldn't beat you here anyway now that you are so healthy again." said Giuliana.

"Well I won either way," said Wesa proudly.

"So, what's the plan?" asked Olivia excitedly. "We've got to have one you know. And a plan B too, that's how they do it in all of the spy movies."

"The plan is this," said Giuliana. "You and Wesa need to cause a diversion while I get setup with Niblet. How about you guys show Professor B how fast Wesa can run. You can race him around the block on your bicycle Olivia. By the time you are finished I will have everything ready for the big moment!"

"And how are we going to get him to sponsor the community gardens and decoder books for the schools?" asked Wesa, still anxious to get started. "Do you really think he is going to do it?"

"I know he will," proclaimed Olivia. "Remember, Niblet

is going to ask him, and besides why wouldn't he. After all, it's a great cause."

"Don't worry Wesa. Professor B will figure out the best way for us to get this project going, that's for sure," Giuliana reassured. "Now, let's go inside. I will tell Professor B that I have to go the bathroom. While I am there, you guys get him to go outside and watch you race. I know how persuasive you can be Olivia."

All the while, Professor B, was curiously watching the kids. He could see they were hatching some type of scheme. What it was, he had no idea, but he thought he would just play along. He was sure it would be fun, but, of course, he was not at all prepared for what was about to unfold.

The kids approached the door, with Giuliana hiding Niblet in her pocket, carrying the computer in her backpack. Olivia rang the doorbell and in no time at all Professor B was standing in the open doorway.

"Good morning sports fans, what are you all doing here so early. The party is not until later." Professor B inquired.

"We were just anxious to come over and help with the decorations and party setup," said Giuliana. "Hey, can I use the bathroom real quick?"

"Of course," said Professor B. "You know where it is."

As Giuliana entered the house, Olivia piped up, "Hey

Wesa, let's race around the block. I will ride my bicycle and you will run. Who do you think will win Professor B?"

"Well, Olivia is pretty fast on her bicycle, but I heard that you are clocking some pretty fast times these days, so, I guess I don't really know," said Professor B.

"You can be the starter Grandpa. Wesa and I will do one lap around the block." Olivia commanded matter-of-factly.

"Got it," said Professor B. "I will officiate."

All the while, Giuliana was in the house firing up the computer and getting everything situated just right. "This was going to be aaaaawwwwesome," she giggled.

Olivia and Wesa took their positions in front of the house, ready to race. Although this was supposed to be a distraction, they both still wanted to win badly and were going to hammer it out.

"On your marks…get…set, GO!" said the professor and off the kids went, Olivia peddling like a Tasmanian devil and Wesa sprinting off just as fast, but a whole lot more gracefully."

Professor B watched as the children sped off and rounded the first corner. As they went out of sight he glanced toward the house and into the bay window. He noticed Giuliana setting up her laptop on the table. "Oh, perhaps they need some help with homework or they are going to show me something they are working on. That must be what this whole charade is about," he thought. "They would never get up this early unless something was afoot."

Within less than a minute the two came tearing around the corner and Professor B stood off of the sidewalk and positioned himself on the lawn so that he could determine the winner. Down the sidewalk they came, sprinting and peddling their little hearts out. The race would come down to the finish. As they approached the finish line, Giuliana looked out the window and said to Niblet, perched on her shoulder, "Look at Wesa now, Niblet. He is strong and healthy and smart again and it's all thanks to you."

Niblet scurried down her arm and jumped onto the table. Sliding around the keypad he replied, "I just did what Professor B trained me for. This is going to be the best birthday present he ever had. All of the work he did was not in vain. His dedication is going to change the world, and today he is going to know it."

In the end, Wesa couldn't beat Olivia on her bicycle, and she gloated plenty. But in fact only Hussein Bolt would have had a chance. Wesa ran like he never had before, it's just that bikes are a whole lot more efficient in transferring energy to velocity than the human body is alone. "I am going to beat you some day," he told Olivia, and he really believed he would.

"Great Race" Shouted Professor B.

"I am the Champion, I am the champion…of the WORLD," sang Olivia in her best Freddy Mercury imitation.

"Well, not exactly "the world" Olivia, but you are the bicycle racing champion of this block, and Wesa is about as fast a person as I have ever seen. Hey, let's go inside and have a snack, then you can tell me what you are really doing here and Giuliana can explain the computer on my kitchen table," said Professor B.

Wesa and Olivia looked at each other coyly. Did Professor B know that they had a game afoot?

"Uh, Ok", said Wesa.

"Sure!" said Olivia.

The kids rushed toward the door as Professor B strolled up the walkway, chuckling to himself about the little show the kids were putting on. They reached the house, pushed open the door and looked quickly at Giuliana and Niblet at the kitchen table. Then, like Meerkats, their heads swiveled back to Professor B and they both smiled insanely at him.

Of the crazy smiles, Professor B took note. "Perhaps there IS more to this than I thought," he mused. "With the kids these days you can never be sure what to expect." Little did he know it was his own work that would be his biggest surprise!

As the Professor entered the house the kids gathered by the table, clearly alluding to the computer, he noticed Niblet doing what looked like a dance on the laptop. "What's going on? What is Niblet doing on the computer?" He exclaimed.

The kids could barely contain themselves but Niblet had finished his first couple of sentences and sent them to the voice synthesizer. "Good Morning, Professor B. I have waited a long time to speak with you. I am sorry about all the trouble I caused you by sending the email to Dr. Johnson. After that I was afraid to speak up fearing I would make it worse. Now I have come forward because we are going to change the world!"

"Why Niblet, you little rascal. I knew that you sent that email. But don't worry about the rest of it. I was ready to shove off from the Company long before the stir that it caused," said the Professor.

"Niblet was the one who taught us about all of chemicals and additives that Wesa was eating and how they were ruining his health. Look at Wesa now. He is better than ever," said Giuliana.

"How long has this been going on? I did notice some strange orders on my account for some software a little while back, I guess I know now what it was for," said Professor B.

"Remember when Niblet got "lost"?" said Olivia.

"Let me explain," said Giuliana.

"Girls, stop the banter. Wesa can explain," said Professor B.

"Ok, so when I moved here from Africa my diet changed completely. I began to eat what my new parents were eating and within several months I was not the same person," said Wesa.

"I can imagine that would be possible." the Professor speculated. "Go On."

"Well, when I met the girls finally in person, they took me to talk to Dad about my health issues," said Wesa. "He suggested that food might be my problem, then told me to read a bunch of books. But the books were way over my head so I was sort of stuck. Giuliana and Olivia wanted to help but they were a bit confused as well. Then I guess Niblet overheard the conversation and decided that he was going to solve the mystery of why I was so sick."

"So, he ran away, hid in the cupboards and studied every night. When he had finished he reappeared and told us exactly what to do." Olivia piped in.

"What do you mean, "Exactly what to do?"" asked the Professor.

"Well, he told us that we had to investigate the foods that Wesa was eating. We actually sort of snuck into his pantry and freezer and took pictures of the labels. Then we took that back to Niblet and he showed us all of the problematic additives and preservatives. After several months of avoiding all of those harmful chemicals and eating only whole foods, my health has improved dramatically," said Wesa.

"He even had us put together a list of the worst additives. And we made a de-coder so that we could share the information with other kids. If it saved Wesa's life, it can certainly help others," said Giuliana.

"Is this all true Niblet?" asked Professor B.

With a whirl Niblet slid around the touchpad, clicking here and there. Soon enough he sent the prose to the voice synthesizer. "All true, Doc. I was certain that this was why you saved from those dreadful experiments at the lab. You know, the ones on the additives that decimated all of my relatives."

"Niblet is AWESOME, Professor B. He really did learn everything that you were trying to teach him. He is Wesa's savior," said Olivia.

"If I wasn't seeing it for myself, even I would not believe it," said Professor B.

"I know, I know," said Wesa. "He helped me so much that I am certain he can do the same for other children."

"Which, I might add, brings us to why we are here," Giuliana added mysteriously.

"Right," Olivia agreed. "We have a plan to Save the World. Remember what Dad always said, "Anything less than changing the world is Mickey Mouse to me?" Well, we are going to change the world, and Niblet is just the one to do it."

"Now wait a minute little ones. How exactly are you planning to "change the world," asked Professor B.

"It is all really very simple," replied Giuliana.

"We are going to print the code books up and send them to all of the schools in the area. Then we are going to convince the school board to hand them out to the children. Finally, we are going to convince them to plant a garden at each school so that the children can produce and enjoy their own real live food," said Wesa.

"And how do you plan to convince the school board to do these things for you?" Professor B inquired.

"That's where you come in Grandpa. We thought you would help us," said Olivia, coyly batting her eyes at Professor B. It was one of the rare times that they called him grandpa and she definitely did it for a reason. They needed his help or they would never accomplish their goals.

"And what exactly am I supposed to do?" Professor B said. "I mean, I am ecstatic by the revelations about Niblet, but I am not going to take him back to the lab and continue his education. I am done with all of that."

"But you are a renowned scientist, and the best gardener I know, so you the perfect person to help. When everyone finds out about your success with Niblet, they will listen to you as never before. All of the stupid rumors will be gone." Giuliana pleaded. "And won't that be nice?"

"Perhaps you are right. I think I have an idea," said the Professor. "Do you remember when Niblet sent that Text to Dr. Johnson? You know, the one that caused so much trouble that I had to resign?"

"Yes, we do. Of course. That is how we got Niblet." Olivia replied.

"It just so happens that Dr. Johnson is on the school board. If we can enlist his support we will be as good as gold," the Professor continued.

"How in the world are you going to get him to help you? Isn't he the one who ran you out of the Company?" said Wesa.

"Yes, he did. But you can't blame him. The evidence pointed to me being a little crazy for believing in Niblet, so he was right to be so critical. But we have since reconciled our differences and I have even invited him over for the party today," the Professor responded.

"I've got a plan," Giuliana interrupted excitedly.

"Yes, and what is it?" said Professor B

"Well, we will make a bet with Dr. Johnson. We'll bet him that if Niblet can talk, he has to promise to help us," Giuliana went on.

"And our wish will be gardens in every school in the district and code books for all of the children as a part of their curriculum," said Wesa.

"That idea has promise," said Professor B. "Dr. Johnson is a good sport. I am certain that he would take the wager. And he has come a long way since our days at the Company and has begun to rethink his former positions on all of these crazy additives."

So, that is how it went. When Dr. Johnson arrived at the party a couple of hours later, he had no idea that his world was about to be turned upside down. But in the end, he proved how good a sport he really was. He couldn't believe his eyes and ears when Niblet started flying around the touchpad and producing audible sentences from the voice synthesizer. At first he thought it was just a ruse, but as the conversation got extremely personal and pointed, Dr. Johnson was forced to admit that Niblet really was a wonder mouse.

"In my wildest imagination I would never have believed this. There is no denying it. Niblet is extraordinary. He can be an amazing catalyst for change. Not only am I going to get those gardens planted, but I am going to personally design a program that Niblet can present himself to the children about food additives. Can you imagine how the children are going to react to a talking scientific mouse?" Dr. Johnson gushed.

"It is going to be Incredible!" shouted Olivia.

"We are going to do it, aren't we?" Wesa said, half in disbelief at the good fortune.

"Fruits and vegetables for all! And no more of those nasty, harmful, chemical concoctions that pass for food. This is the beginning of a new chapter. We have the knowledge and the support to make a difference and we are going to make it happen," said Giuliana.

10 TIMES HAVE CHANGED

Professor B finished the book, closed it and placed it on his lap. He took off his glasses and rubbed his eyes. Wow, what a story. Two little girls, an African boy and a talking mouse really had changed the world, or at least, they had changed their world. Wesa was healthy and thriving, and his parents were too. The schools now had community gardens and the children were learning about harmful additives in the classroom. What a change from just a few years ago when Professor B has left the Company in disgust.

He got up from his chair and went back to the window. He looked down at the peppers, tomatoes and all of the other produce in the garden. Even the University had allowed them to plant a garden on campus. This whole scenario really had created a historical rupture that changed the future.

Meanwhile, he thought, after getting so much attention in the community, Niblet and the kids had garnered national praise for their efforts and had been invited to the White House to receive a special award for their efforts. The first lady was so overwhelmed by their work on the gardens that she had decided to put one in on the White House lawn.

He still could not believe it, but he knew it was true. How proud he was of those kids and especially that mouse. They had followed their heart and had worked selflessly to help their friends and then the whole community. Countless lives had been affected by their efforts and he knew that it was only the beginning. After all these were just children. Imagine what they would be capable of when they grew up!

Not the End: The Beginning

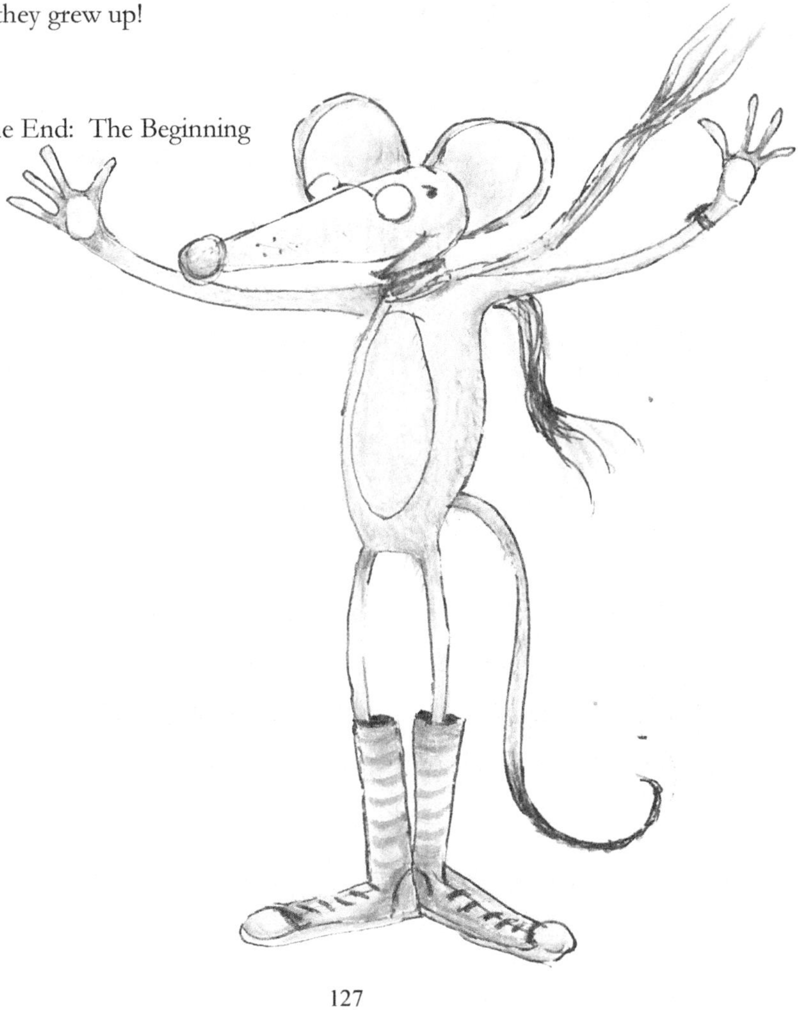

De-Coder List of Problem Ingredients

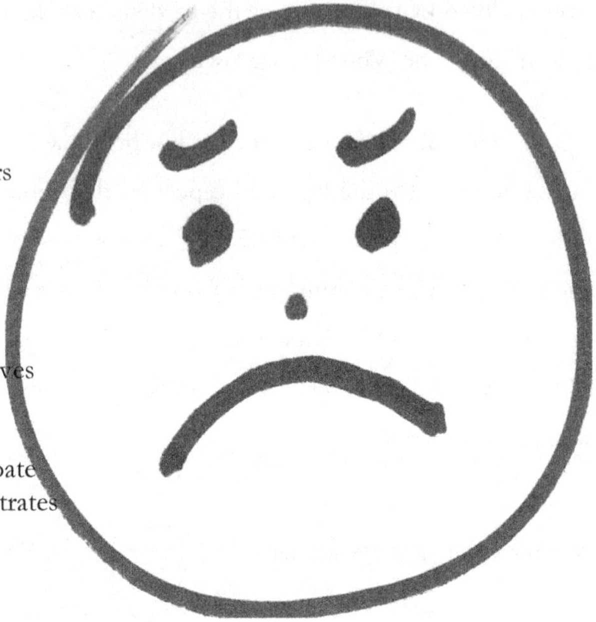

Artificial Colors

Artificial Flavors

All Artificial Sweeteners
- Aspartame
- Acelfame K
- Sucralose
- Splenda

All Artificial Perservatives
- BHT, BHA
- TBHQ
- Sodium Benzoate
- Nitites and Nitrates

Free Glutamates

Hyrolyzed Protein

Enriched or other Non Whole Grain Flours

High Fructose Corn Syrup and any other added Sugars

Hyrdrogenated Oils

Non Organic Soy Proteins

Genetically Modified Foods (All non-organic Corn and Soy)

Read the ingredients panel. Write a Sad face every time you see any of the additives or ingredients above. Write a happy face when you see a real whole food item. Then compare how many happy to sad faces you have and decide whether to eat something. GO TO WWW.CHEMICALFREELUNCH.COM TO KNOW MORE!

IF YOU DON'T READ IT – YOU SHOULDN'T EAT IT!

ABOUT THE AUTHOR

Marshall Carder is a true renaissance man. He graduated from the University of California San Diego in political science, working his way through. He received little help from his parents who still lived in the community where he grew up. After college he worked for a year saved his money, and left for Europe to learn about the world. Several months later he met his wife to be, a young woman from Brazil who was on holiday in Germany. He traveled to Rio to join her, staying for six months. He became fluent in Brazilian Portuguese and first saw the art of Capoeira, the Brazilian martial art. He and Ana returned to the US, married, and have two children. Marshall has a very broad arsenal of skills. He is a carpenter, a plumber, an expert in Brazilian martial arts, an excellent chef (A good cook can prepare an excellent meal for family and friends. A chef can feed a multitude), a golfer with a five handicap, a businessman, an accomplished salesperson, and most relevant to this book, an outstanding father to two daughters, a fluent writer, and a committed student of nutrition.

Made in the USA
Monee, IL
04 November 2026

67377656R00075